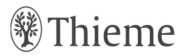

Pocket Atlas of Spine Surgery

Second Edition

Kern Singh, MD
Professor
Department of Orthopaedic Surgery
Co-Director, Minimally Invasive Spine Institute
Rush University Medical Center
Chicago, Illinois

Alexander R. Vaccaro, MD, PhD
Richard H. Rothman Professor and Chairman
Department of Orthopaedic Surgery
Professor of Neurosurgery
Thomas Jefferson University and Hospitals
President, The Rothman Institute
Philadelphia, Pennsylvania

201 illustrations

Thieme
New York • Stuttgart • Delhi • Rio de Janeiro

Executive Editor: William Lamsback
Managing Editor: Nikole Y. Connors
Director, Editorial Services: Mary Jo Casey
Production Editor: Naamah Schwartz
International Production Director: Andreas Schabert
Editorial Director: Sue Hodgson
International Marketing Director: Fiona Henderson
International Sales Director: Louisa Turrell
Director of Institutional Sales: Adam Bernacki
Senior Vice President and Chief Operating Officer:
Sarah Vanderbilt
President: Brian D. Scanlan

Illustrations drawn by Andrea Hines

Library of Congress Cataloging-in-Publication Data

Names: Singh, Kern, author. | Vaccaro, Alexander R.,
author.
Title: Pocket atlas of spine surgery / Kern Singh,
Alexander R. Vaccaro.
Description: Second edition. | New York : Thieme, [2018]
| Includes
  bibliographical references.
Identifiers: LCCN 2017046568| ISBN 9781626236233
(print) | ISBN 9781626236240
  (e-book)
Subjects: | MESH: Spine--surgery | Atlases | Handbooks
Classification: LCC RD768 | NLM WE 17 | DDC
617.4/71--dc23 LC record available at https://lccn.loc.
gov/2017046568

© 2018 Thieme Medical Publishers, Inc.

Thieme Publishers New York
333 Seventh Avenue, New York, NY 10001 USA
+1 800 782 3488, customerservice@thieme.com

Thieme Publishers Stuttgart
Rüdigerstrasse 14, 70469 Stuttgart, Germany
+49 [0]711 8931 421, customerservice@thieme.de

Thieme Publishers Delhi
A-12, Second Floor, Sector-2, Noida-201301
Uttar Pradesh, India
+91 120 45 566 00, customerservice@thieme.in

Thieme Publishers Rio de Janeiro, Thieme Publicações
Ltda.
Edifício Rodolpho de Paoli, 25º andar
Av. Nilo Peçanha, 50 – Sala 2508,
Rio de Janeiro 20020-906 Brasil
+55 21 3172-2297 / +55 21 3172-1896

Cover design: Thieme Publishing Group
Typesetting by DiTech Process Solutions

Printed in Germany by Beltz Grafische Betriebe,
Bad Langensalza   5 4 3 2 1

ISBN 978-1-62623-623-3

Also available as an e-book:
eISBN 978-1-62623-624-0

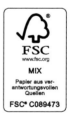

I dedicate this book to my father. As I now progress into parenthood, I realize the sacrifices you made for me. Never ending patience, bountiful amounts of time, and a dedication to giving me every opportunity to succeed.

- K. Singh

This book is dedicated to my one and only true hero, my father, Alexander Vaccaro, Sr., who to this day I look to for guidance and wisdom in all aspects of my life.

- A. Vaccaro

Contents

Foreword

Alex Vaccaro and Kern Singh are friends of mine, colleagues, and inspirational spine surgeons that have put their passion together to bring us *Pocket Atlas of Spine Surgery, 2nd edition*. While I have known both for many years and learned a great deal from their experience and view of spine surgery, it should be a pleasant surprise to readers that this book brings their divergent perspectives into a concise and practical publication.

Pocket Atlas of Spine Surgery, 2nd edition offers spine surgeons a unique and efficient guide to surgical techniques. Through excellent visual guides and anatomic overlay the relevant anatomy of key procedures is elegantly portrayed. The step-by-step descriptions concisely present anatomical considerations, and tips every surgeon can employ. In the summary portion of each paragraph is highly relevant content related to potential complications and suggested reading.

I congratulate Alex and Kern on their fine work and valuable contribution to our field. This book is a 'must have' for every spine surgeon and a real pleasure to read and learn from.

Frank Schwab, MD
Chief, Spine Service
Hospital for Special Surgery
Professor of Orthopaedic Surgery
Weill Cornell Medical College
New York, New York

Preface

This spine surgery atlas was created as a pocket-friendly resource that practicing medical professionals can bring right into the operating room with them. The detailed illustrations that overlay high quality intraoperative photos allow the reader to visualize the entire surgical field, including the anatomy that is never "seen" while operating. This translucent view into complex spinal anatomy helps the reader understand the subtleties of technically demanding techniques such as minimally invasive spinal surgery. This artwork allows the reader to become comfortable with the surgery before setting foot in the operating room. The accompanying text not only describes the surgical technique, but also offers pearls and tips to help perform the procedure expeditiously. Common complications are described, as well as suggestions for their avoidance.

The second edition provides several additional advantages. The text has been enhanced with new images, including cross-sectional illustrations to further describe surgical approaches and radiographs that demonstrate postoperative results. Further emphasis has been provided on superficial landmarks, potential pitfalls, and common complications. This allows for improved mastery of the surgical procedures and postoperative care. Finally, the text has been updated based on current knowledge in the rapidly advancing field of spine surgery and includes suggestions for additional readings.

This atlas will serve as a valuable resource not only for orthopedic surgeons, neurosurgeons, and surgical trainees such as residents and fellows, but also for physician assistants, nursing staff personnel, and anyone else involved in the operative care of spine surgery patients. We hope this atlas will provide readers with an improved understanding of the intricacies of spinal surgery.

Acknowledgments

We would like to thank all of those who assisted in the creation of this book. In particular, we would like to acknowledge Brittany Haws and Benjamin Khechen for their efforts in seeing this book to completion.

1 Anterior Cervical Diskectomy and Fusion

■ Anterior Cervical Positioning

- Removal of cervical disk herniations
- Removal of uncinate osteophytes
- Cervical interbody fusions
- Removal of tumors
- Treatment of infection and abscesses

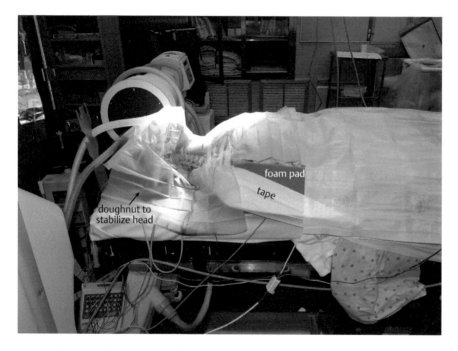

- The head is placed onto a doughnut to maintain its position. A bump or roll is placed horizontally across the scapulae to allow for gentle extension of the cervical spine. Care should be taken to avoid hyperextension in patients with spinal cord compression and myelopathy. Tape is applied to the top of the shoulders to depress them gently for improved visualization of the lower cervical segments. A foam pad is placed over the elbows to protect the ulnar nerve.

Tips and Pearls before You Begin

Anatomic landmarks may aid in the placement of the surgical incision. Typically, the hyoid bone overlies the C3 vertebral body, the thyroid cartilage overlies the C4–C5 intervertebral disk space, and the cricoid ring overlies the C6 level. Disk space localization is performed with a radiopaque marker and a lateral radiograph. Needles for localization should be placed into the vertebral body and not the disk space to prevent possible disk degeneration in case the wrong level is localized.

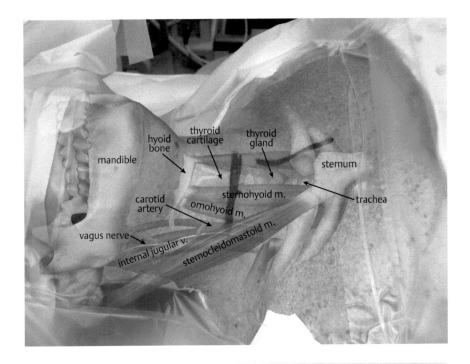

Superficial landmarks include:

- Lower border of mandible: C2–C3
- Hyoid bone: C3
- Thyroid cartilage: C4–C5
- Cricoid cartilage: C6

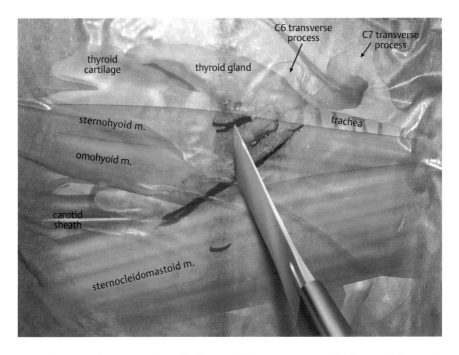

- A horizontal incision is made just medial to the sternocleidomastoid muscle (SCM).
- A decision on a right- or left-side approach should be made based on surgeon comfort.

Internervous Plane

No internervous plane is present during this superficial dissection. The platysma muscle directly beneath the fascial sheath will be incised with the skin. It is innervated by branches of the facial nerve superiorly.

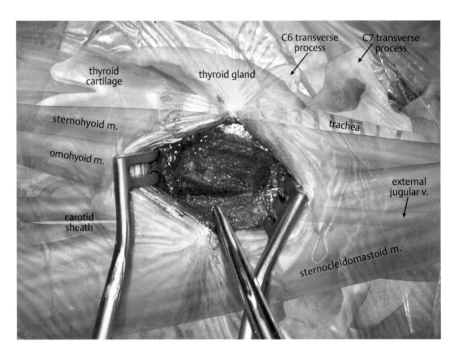

- The platysma is divided in line with the skin incision.
- The external jugular vein helps to identify the tracheoesophageal groove.

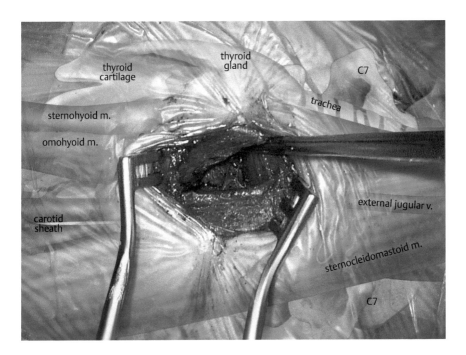

- The SCM and carotid sheath are retracted laterally:
  - The carotid sheath contains:
    - Internal jugular vein
    - Carotid artery
    - Vagus nerve
- The tracheoesophageal complex is retracted medially:
  - Sternohyoid, sternothyroid strap muscles, and thyroid retracted medially as well.
  - The recurrent laryngeal nerve lies in the tracheoesophageal groove.

Potential Pitfalls

Carotid sheath is protected by anterior border of SCM. Placing self-retaining retractors when dissecting laterally may endanger its contents.

Internervous Plane

An internervous plane is present between the SCM (cranial nerve XI—spinal accessory nerve) and strap muscles (C1, C2, C3).

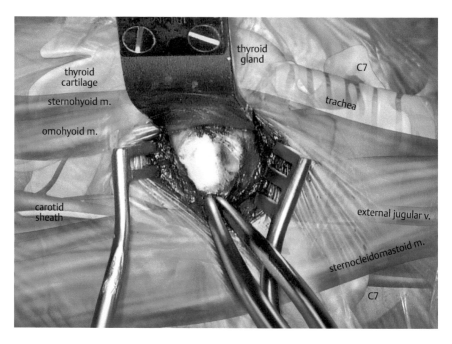

- The longus colli are swept laterally, exposing the superficial disk space.
- A knife or electrocautery device can be used to perform the annulotomy.

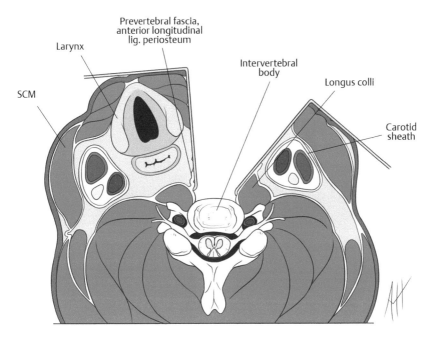

Cross section. SCM and carotid sheath are retracted laterally, and tracheoesophogeal complex is retracted medially. Longus colli is removed subperiosteally from vertebral body, exposing the intervertebral disk and anterior surface of vertebral body.

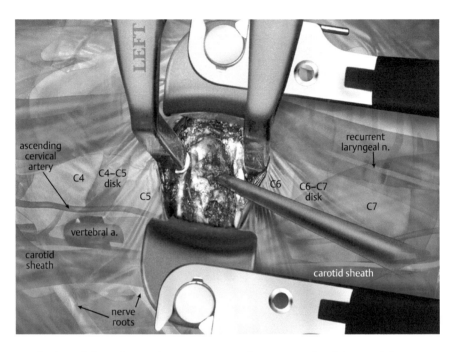

- Both straight and curved curettes are used to remove the disk material.
- Caspar pins are used to distract the disk space and to improve visualization of the posterior intervertebral space.

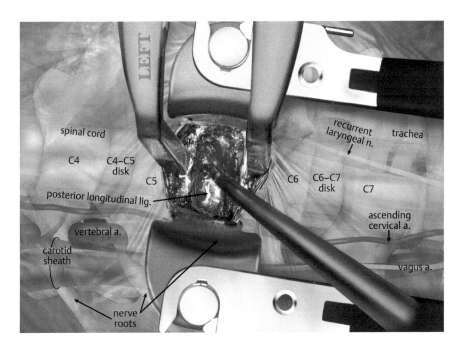

- A microcurette or nerve hook, along with a 1-mm Kerrison rongeur, can be used to remove the posterior longitudinal ligament:
  – A 6–0 angled curette is helpful for getting behind the uncinate process.

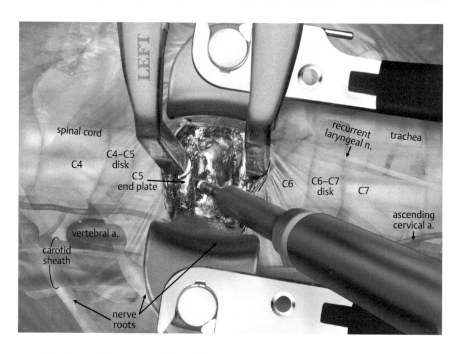

- A high-speed burr is used for a decortication of the end plates:
  - The burr is also used to create parallel end plates to improve contact between the bone graft and the end plate.

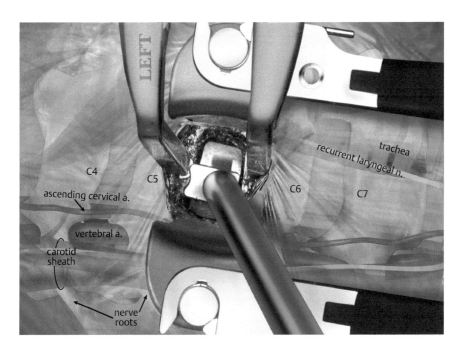

• A trial sizer is placed to approximate the intervertebral space.

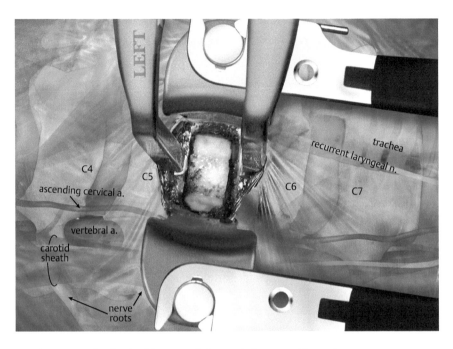

- An appropriately sized bone graft is gently impacted into place.
  - The Caspar pins are removed to allow compression across the graft:
    - Bone wax is placed into the Caspar pin holes to control bleeding.

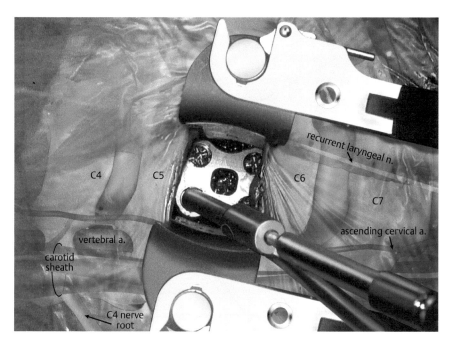

- An anterior cervical plate is applied.
  - The shortest feasible plate should be used to avoid abutment of the adjacent disk space.

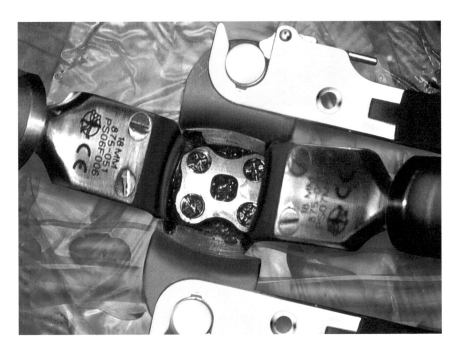

- Cervical screws that typically measure 12 to 16 mm are placed through the plate.
- Depending on the preference of the surgeon, fixed or variable screws may be used to allow for controlled subsidence.

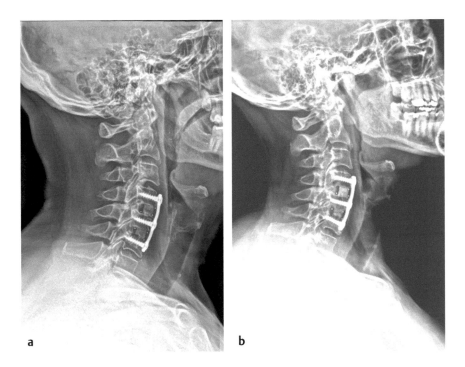

a

b

Postoperative radiographs: **(a)** Six weeks postoperatively, with evidence of successful screw placement. **(b)** Six months postoperatively, showing solid fusion.

Perioperative Complications

- **Horner's Syndrome:**
  - Damage or irritation to the **sympathetic nerves or stellate ganglion.**
  - Characterized by ptosis, anhydrosis, miosis, and loss of ciliospinal reflex.
  - Prevention:
    - Place retractors under medial edge of longus colli during periosteal dissection.
- **Hoarseness:**
  - Damage to the recurrent laryngeal nerve:
    - **Left recurrent laryngeal nerve**—originates at the aortic arch and ascends between the trachea and esophagus.
    - **Right recurrent laryngeal nerve**—originates at the right subclavian artery, passes from lateral to medial towards the tracheoesophageal groove.
  - Prevention:
    - Place retractors under medial edge of longus colli.
- **Dysphagia:**
  - Overzealous retraction of esophagus.
  - Risk factors:
    - Increased retraction time
    - Upper cervical dissection (C3-C4 or proximal)
    - Patients with preoperative dysphagia
    - Female sex
  - Prevention:
    - Intermittent relaxation of self-retaining retractors during the procedure and partially deflating the endotracheal cuff once the cervical retractors are in position
- **Retropharyngeal hematoma:**
  - Development of postsurgical edema and bleeding.
  - Characterized by respiratory difficulties and tense mass under incision.
  - Prevention:
    - Placement of surgical drain
    - Consider for those with older age, history of smoking, and increased operative levels
  - Treatment:
    - Emergent decompression
- **Pseudarthrosis:**
  - Failure of interbody fusion
  - Risk factors:
    - Increased operative levels
    - Smoking
    - Diabetes

■ Suggested Readings

1. Singh K, Marquez-Lara A, Nandyala SV, Patel AA, Fineberg SJ. Incidence and risk factors for dysphagia after anterior cervical fusion. Spine 2013;38(21):1820–1825
2. Riley LH III, Vaccaro AR, Dettori JR, Hashimoto R. Postoperative dysphagia in anterior cervical spine surgery. Spine 2010;35(9, Suppl):S76–S85
3. Basques BA, Bohl DD, Golinvaux NS, Yacob A, Varthi AG, Grauer JN. Factors predictive of increased surgical drain output after anterior cervical discectomy and fusion. Spine 2014;39(9):728–735
4. Stachniak JB, Diebner JD, Brunk ES, Speed SM. Analysis of prevertebral soft-tissue swelling and dysphagia in multilevel anterior cervical discectomy and fusion with recombinant human bone morphogenetic protein-2 in patients at risk for pseudarthrosis. J Neurosurg Spine 2011;14(2):244–249

2 Anterior Cervical Corpectomy and Fusion

Obtaining proper imaging studies is paramount for optimal surgical treatment. Careful evaluation of the location and course of the **vertebral artery** is necessary to avoid iatrogenic injury. At the time of surgery, complete diskectomies before resection of the vertebral bodies facilitate assessment of the depth of the vertebral body as well as the location of the spinal canal. In cases where an **ossified posterior longitudinal ligament** (PLL) is extremely adherent to the **dura**, direct resection can be dangerous. Successful decompression can be performed by removing the PLL on either side of the ossified area and allowing it to float away anteriorly from the cord (anterior floating technique) without necessitating direct resection. When a corpectomy is performed, a high-speed burr can be used to resect most of the vertebral body, leaving only a thin rim of posterior cortical bone. The posterior cortical bone can be removed using either a small curette or a Kerrison rongeur.

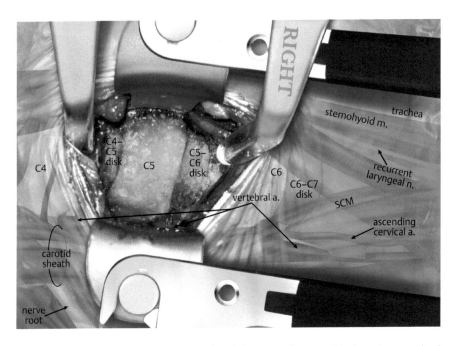

- Before the corpectomy is begun, the disk space above and below the vertebral body to be resected is clearly exposed.
- The uncovertebral margin is the most reliable reference in determining the lateral extent of the vertebral body resection.
  - A Penfield elevator may be used to palpate the transverse process to ensure that lateral dissection is sufficient.
    - The vertebral artery lies deeper than the plane of dissection (posterior middle third of the vertebral body).

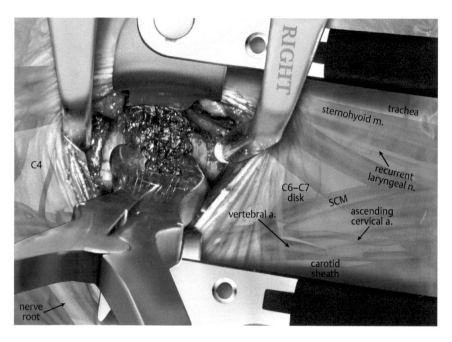

- A Leksell rongeur can be used to remove most of the vertebral body quickly.

Potential Pitfalls

Vertebral artery injury can occur with extensive lateral decompression. The vertebral artery is located within the transverse foramen of vertebrae C3–C6.

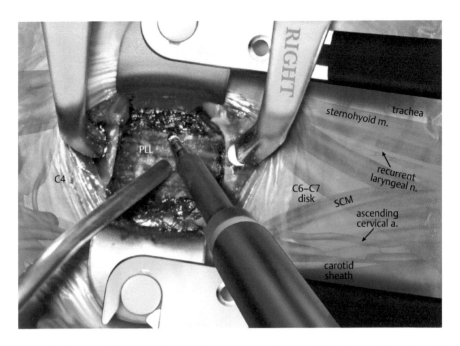

- A high-speed burr can be used to remove the remaining bone laterally and posteriorly until the PLL is identified:
  - In most cases, an adequate decompression can be accomplished while preserving the PLL, which can then serve to prevent overdistraction from the interposed graft:
    - The defect should be widened to the uncovertebral margin to ensure adequate thecal sac decompression.

Potential Pitfalls

The PLL is occasionally noted to be severely adherent to the dura, causing thecal sac manipulation and spinal cord constriction. Intraoperative dural tears can occur during removal of the posterior vertebral body and PLL in these instances.

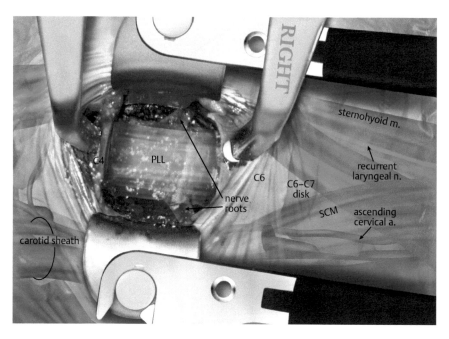

- Bleeding from the cancellous vertebral body can be controlled with Gelfoam or other thrombotic agents.

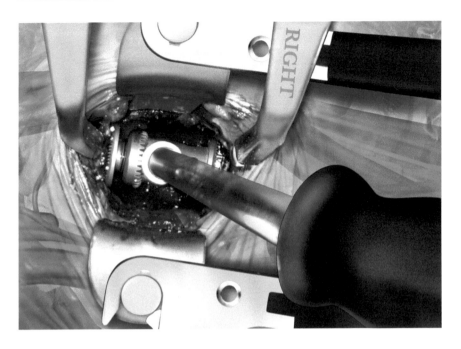

- The exposed end plates can be used to determine an appropriate size for the cage or graft.
- If an expandable cage is used, expansion should be performed with lateral fluoroscopy to prevent overdistraction.

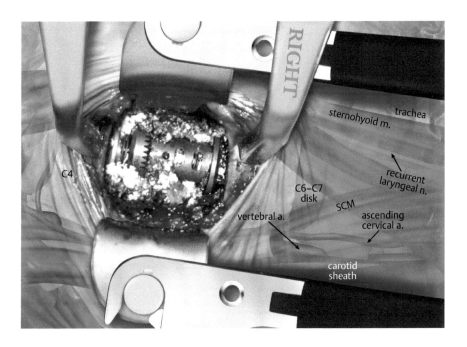

- The bone graft from the corpectomy site can be placed into and around the cage:
  - Bone should be saved in nonneoplastic or noninfectious cases.
  - In cases of malignancy or infection, bone graft substitute should be utilized.

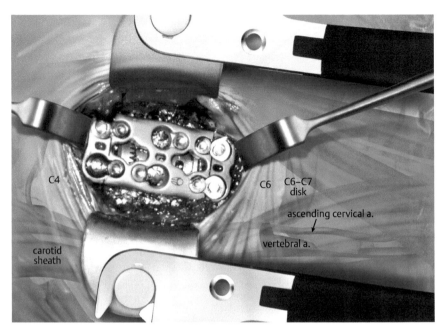

- A plate can then secure the cage and graft in place:
  - Posterior supplementation should be considered in cases of poor bone quality or in multilevel corpectomies:
    - Posterior supplementation increases fusion rate in two- and three-level corpectomies.

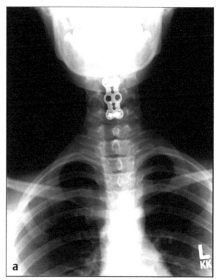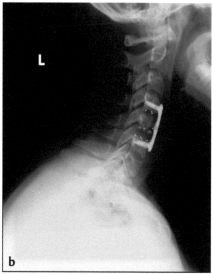

Postoperative radiographs. The patient suffered a traumatic C5 burst fracture with neurological deficit. Anteroposterior **(a)** and lateral **(b)** radiographs demonstrate C5 corpectomy (PEEK [polyetheretherketone] cage) with an anterior cervical plate extending from C4 to C6.

Perioperative Complications[a]

- **Vertebral artery injury:**
  - Transection of the vertebral artery due to extensive lateral decompression or anatomical arterial variants
  - Presents with hemorrhage and possible acute central nervous system ischemia
  - Treatment:
    - Aggressive intravenous fluid resuscitation
    - Placement of the head in a neutral position
    - Hemostasis via digital pressure, Gelfoam
    - Definitive surgical intervention: primary repair, bypass, or sacrifice:
      ○ Nondominant vertebral artery can be sacrificed without complication.
  - Prevention:
    - Evaluation of arterial course on preoperative imaging
- **Intraoperative dural tear, cerebrospinal fluid (CSF) leak, or neurologic injury:**
  - Occurs from excessive dissection of the posterior vertebral body and PLL
  - Characterized by orthostatic headache, nausea, and vomiting
  - Treatment:
    - Patch the defect with collagen matrix or tissue allograft.
    - Apply fibrin glue or sealant
    - Consider lumbar drain to divert CSF
- **Graft dislodgement/instrumentation failure:**
  - Occurs secondary to pseudoarthrosis, infection, prior posterior decompressive procedures, multilevel corpectomy
  - Presents acutely with possible tracheal compression
  - Treatment:
    - Airway stabilization with emergent intubation if significant tracheal compression present
    - Revision with a posterior stabilizing procedure to adequately protect the anterior construct

[a]For complications of anterior approach, see Perioperative Complications in **Chapter 1: Anterior Cervical Diskectomy and Fusion**.

3 Open Posterior Cervical Foraminotomy

Posterior Cervical Positioning

- Removal of paracentral/foraminal cervical disk herniations
- Expansion of spinal canal through laminectomy or laminoplasty
- Removal of spinal cord tumors
- Reduction of facet joint dislocations or fractures
- Posterior spinal fusion for trauma and degenerative cervical conditions

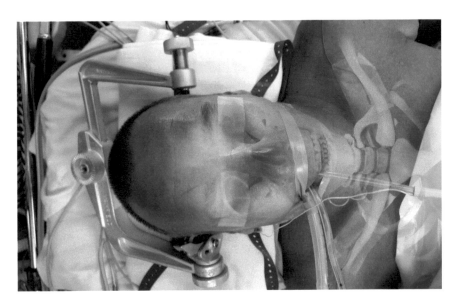

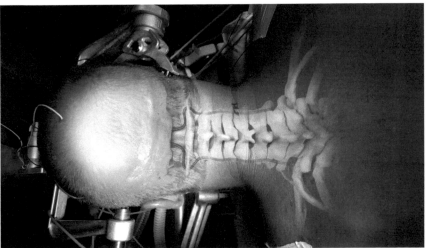

• The Mayfield is placed with the pins along the mastoid process and posterior to the temporal artery and masseter muscle. The pins are typically tightened to 60 to 80 psi.

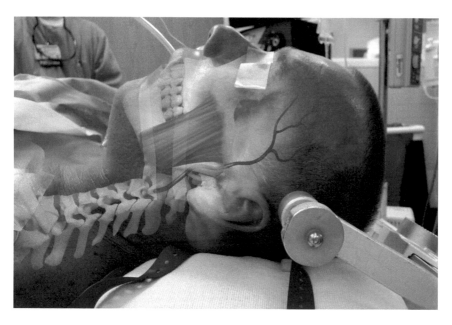

- The table is slightly raised with the head above the feet (reverse Trendelenburg) to allow for venous drainage.

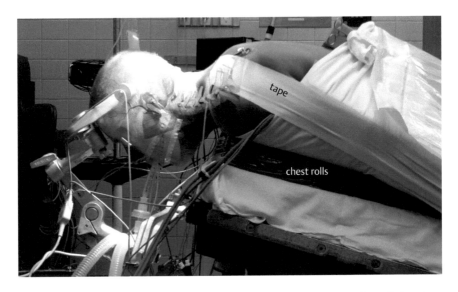

• The patient is then placed into a prone position with chest rolls and the May-field locked into the operative position. Flexion of the neck allows for opening of the spinal canal and easier decompression. A more neutral alignment should be performed prior to placement of the final instrumentation. The arms are gently taped with a gentle depression of the shoulders to allow for increased visualization of the lower cervical segments.

Superficial landmarks include:

– Lower border of mandible: C2–C3
– Hyoid bone: C3
– Thyroid cartilage: C4–C5
– Cricoid cartilage: C6

Tips and Pearls before You Begin

Intraoperative imaging is mandatory to confirm the correct level of decompression. The use of anatomic landmarks can be helpful in many cases, but normal anatomic variants may lead to confusion and ultimately to surgery on the wrong level. Placing a radiopaque marker (such as a needle) into the spinous process at the pathologic level can be helpful. Visualization can be enhanced with an operating microscope or with a combination of loupes and a fiberoptic headlight.

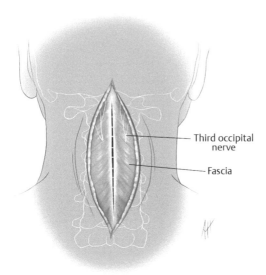

- A straight incision is made midline over the designated pathologic level:
  - The previously placed needle or marker can be used as a guide and center for the incision
- The incision is continued until reaching the spinal processes through the nuchal ligament.

Internervous Plane

The internervous plane is located at midline of the neck between the paraspinal cervical muscles of either side. The dorsal rami of the cervical roots supply the motor and sensory innervation in this region.

Note: A dorsal ramus can occasionally be cauterized with no clinical effect due to redundant innervation.

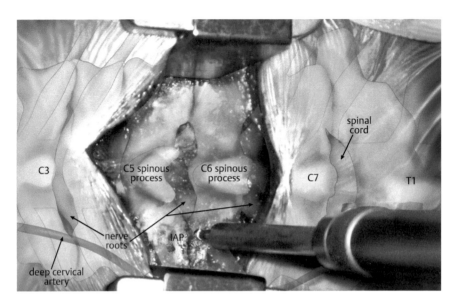

- The paracervical muscles are removed subperiosteally from the posterior cervical vertebrae until lamina and facet joints are revealed:
  - A Cobb elevator or cautery can be used to dissect the muscle without causing unnecessary trauma.
  - The muscles can be removed unilaterally or bilaterally depending on the intended procedure.
- The inferior articular process (IAP) of the cephalad vertebra is identified.

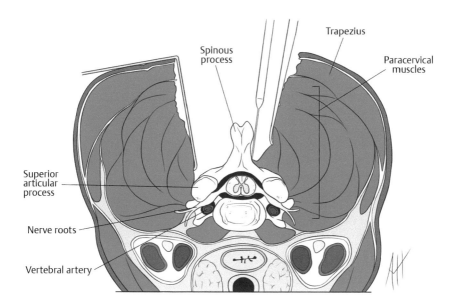

Cross section. Paracervical spinal muscles are removed unilaterally. The vertebral artery is located anterior to the facet joints and nerve roots.

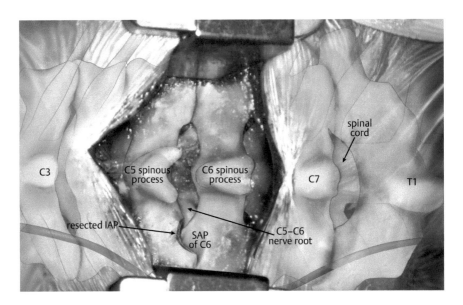

- Approximately 35% of the medial portion of the IAP is removed to visualize the superior articular process (SAP) of the caudal vertebra.

Potential Pitfalls

Cervical instability can occur from excessive removal of the facet joint. No more than 50% of the facet should be removed.

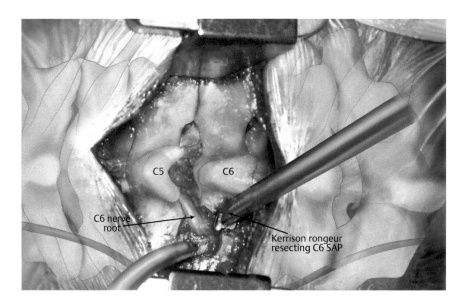

• A Kerrison rongeur or burr can be used to resect the SAP, which overlies the exiting nerve root.

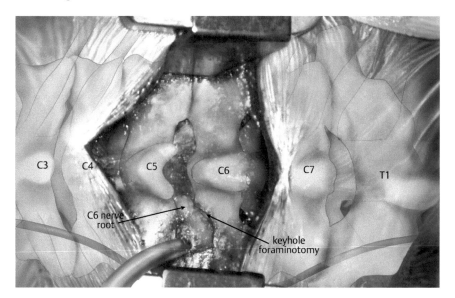

Potential Pitfalls

Free disk material underneath the nerve root can be removed from this exposure. Care should be taken to avoid excessive **nerve root** retraction or dural manipulation.

Perioperative Complications

- **Secondary instability:**
  - Excision of more than 50% of the facet:
    - Torsional stiffness of the cervical spine becomes compromised.
  - Prevention:
    - Remove approximately 30 to 35% of facet joint.
    - To minimize facet excision, work inferior to nerve root during facet removal. Once larger space is achieved, remove the rim immediately dorsal to the nerve root.
- **Cerebrospinal fluid leak:**
  - Dural tear during disk removal:
    - Patients with **spina bifida** are at increased risk for dural and neural tissue damage
    - Infrequent complication (0.6–2.5%)
  - Prevention:
    - Increase exposure size to avoid excessive nerve traction during herniation excision
- **Intraoperative bleeding/postoperative hematoma:**
  - Thin-walled epidural vessels in the cervical canal.
  - Treatment:
    - Control bleeding with hemostatic sponges (such as Gelfoam or bipolar cautery)
    - Placement of wound drains usually not routinely necessary

Suggested Readings

1. Zdeblick TA, Zou D, Warden KE, McCabe R, Kunz D, Vanderby R. Cervical stability after foraminotomy. A biomechanical in vitro analysis. J Bone Joint Surg Am 1992;74(1):22–27
2. Jagannathan J, Sherman JH, Szabo T, Shaffrey CI, Jane JA. The posterior cervical foraminotomy in the treatment of cervical disc/osteophyte disease: a single-surgeon experience with a minimum of 5 years' clinical and radiographic follow-up. J Neurosurg Spine 2009;10(4):347–356

4 Minimally Invasive Posterior Cervical Foraminotomy

A minimally invasive cervical foraminotomy potentially reduces operative time, blood loss, hospital length of stay, and postoperative pain when compared to the open equivalent. However, as in the open posterior cervical foraminotomy, minimally invasive cervical foraminotomy requires intraoperative imaging to confirm the correct level of decompression. The use of anatomic landmarks can be helpful in many cases, but normal anatomic variants may cause confusion and ultimately lead to surgery on the wrong level. In addition, preoperative imaging should be evaluated for a potential anomalous vertebral artery course. Presence of an aberrant vertebral artery may alter surgical planning in order to avoid injury, hemorrhage, and cerebral ischemia.

Superficial landmarks include:

- Spinous processes:
    - C2, C7, and C1 are the largest spinous processes in the region:
        - C7 and T1 are difficult to distinguish from each other
    - Distance between facet joints are extremely small

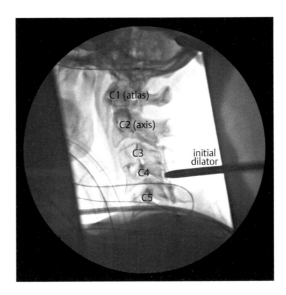

- A lateral fluoroscopic image is used to identify the level in question.
- An incision is made 0.5 cm lateral to the midline.

Internervous Plane

No true internervous plane is present in this procedure; the entry points are within the paraspinal muscles, which are segmentally innervated.

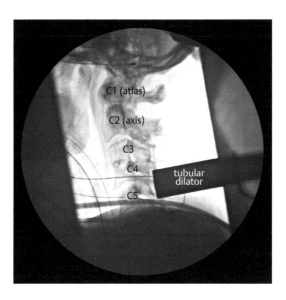

• Tubular dilators (18 mm) are used to spread the paraspinal muscles.

Internervous Plane

Muscle creep can occur with inaccurate placement of tubular dilators. Adequate use of fluoroscopy is necessary to ensure proper dilator positioning.

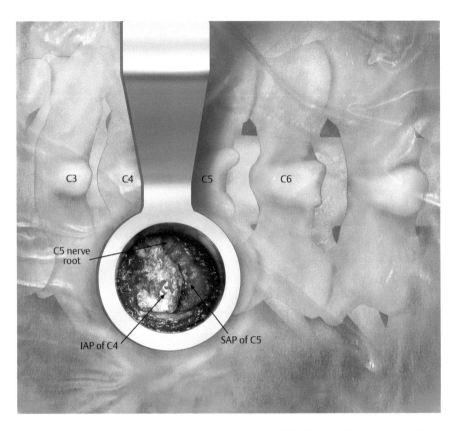

- The soft tissue is removed, exposing the medial half of the facet joint and the inferior portion of the superior lamina.

Potential Pitfalls

Avoid dissection lateral to the facet joint in order to preserve as much of the facet capsule as possible. Furthermore, injury to the **epidural venous plexus** can lead to unnecessary bleeding.

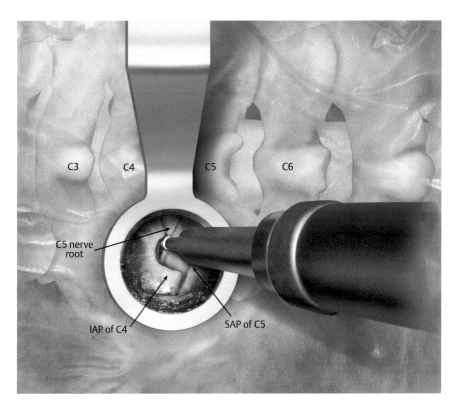

- A burr is used to remove the medial third of the inferior articular process of the cephalad vertebrae.

Potential Pitfalls

Excessive **nerve root retraction** can lead to focal neurologic deficits. Avoid excessive retraction by drilling into the superomedial quadrant of the caudad pedicle to allow improved access to the disk space.

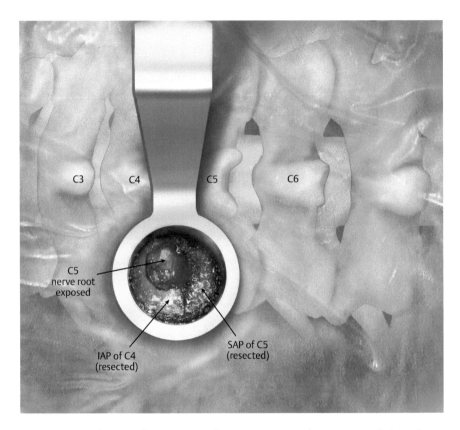

- A burr is then used to remove the superior articular process of the inferior vertebrae.
- The nerve root is then visualized exiting into the neuroforamen.

Potential Pitfalls

Instability can occur from excessive removal of bone from the facet joints. No more than 50% of the facet should be removed.

Perioperative Complications

See **Chapter 3: Open Posterior Cervical Foraminotomy** for common complications also occurring after a minimally invasive cervical foraminotomy

5 Posterior Laminoplasty with Instrumentation

Incise the nuchal ligament and paracervical muscles at the exact midline, and strip the muscles subperiosteally to avoid bleeding. Be careful not to strip or expose the cervical facet capsules. Complete the hinge-side gutter following the completion of the open-side gutter and the resection of the ligamentum flavum at both ends of the laminar door. Check the stability of the hinge frequently while making the hinge gutter; this allows the ability to preserve tension on the opening door. Preserve the spinous process of C7 whenever possible to reduce postoperative axial symptoms. Encourage early active range of motion of the neck.

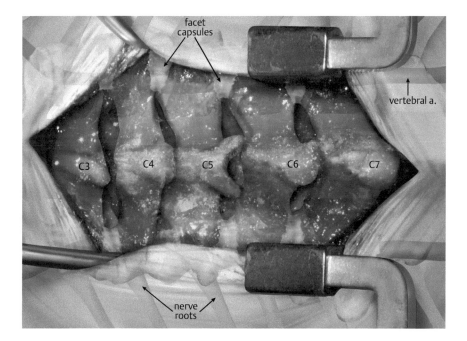

- A midline posterior cervical exposure is performed.
- Care is taken not to strip the facet capsule.
- Only the medial portion of the lamina/facet junction is exposed.

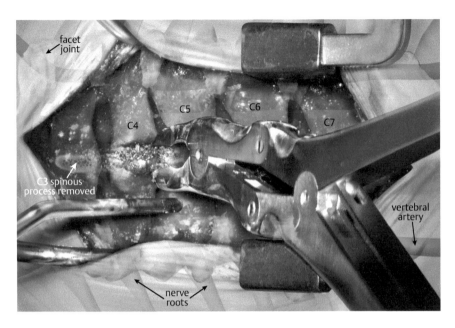

- Once exposed, the spinous processes from C3–C7 are removed.

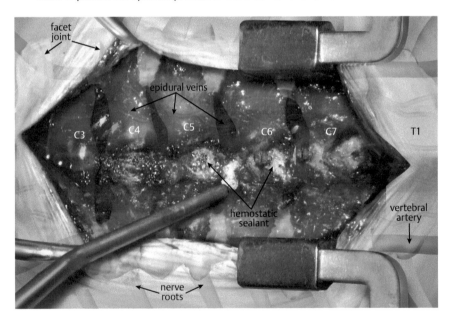

- Once the spinous processes are removed, bone wax or a hemostatic sealant is applied to control bone bleeding.
- The junction between the lamina and facet is identified.

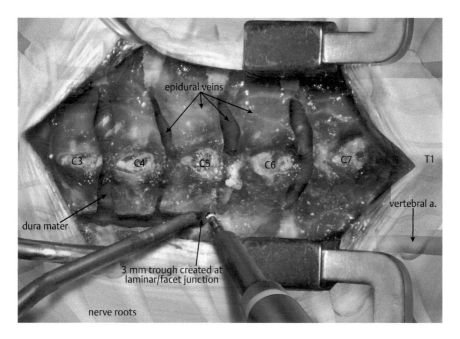

- A burr is used to create an opening of approximately 3 mm.
- This opening requires the removal of 15% of the facet joint.

Potential Pitfalls

Facet joint disruption can occur with drilling lateral to the lamina–facet junction. Direct the drill medially to avoid excessive joint removal.

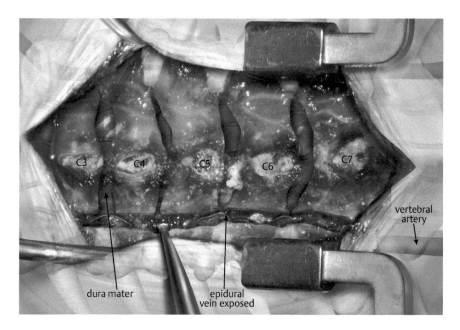

- Once the opening is through the lamina, the epidural veins overlying the dura are visualized.
- A curved microcurette can be used to palpate the defect to ensure that the trough is through the bone.

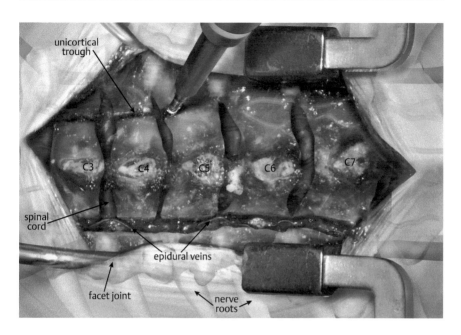

- Once the first trough is complete, a similar trough is created on the other side (hinge side):
  - However, the hinge side is only **unicortical**.

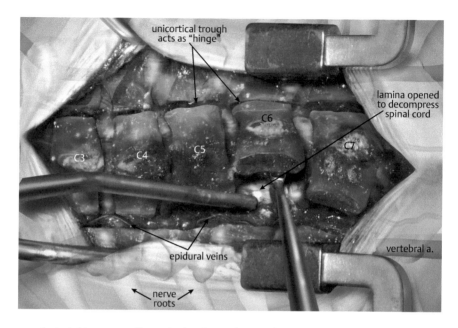

- A straight curette allows the lamina to be gently opened like a door.
- The spinal cord is then gently decompressed and allowed to float back dorsally once the laminae are opened.
- Small 10- to 14-mm craniofacial plates are applied on the opening side.

Potential Pitfalls

Laminar fracture can occur if inadequate amount of drilling is performed on the hinge side. Lift gently and ensure both outer cortex and some cancellous bone have been drilled to avoid a true fracture.

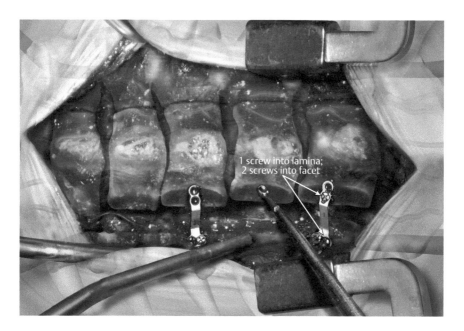

- The plates are secured with 5-mm screws:
  - Two are fastened into the lateral mass
  - One is fastened into the lamina (if necessary)
- The plate secures the lamina in an expanded state, decompressing the spinal cord.

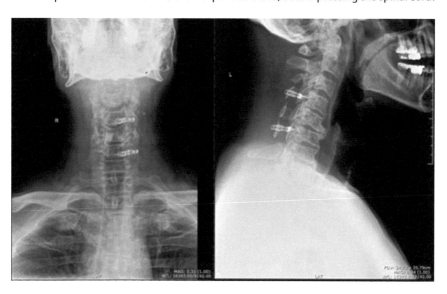

Postoperative radiographs. Postoperative radiographs of a patient with a C3–C6 posterior cervical laminoplasty with instrumentation.

Perioperative Complications

- **C5 nerve palsy:**
  - Incidence of 0.5 to 13.3%
  - Unclear etiology; potentially due to posterior translation of spinal cord and subsequent stretching of the short C5 nerve root, or possible extradural tethering effect.
  - Characterized by deltoid and biceps weakness, sensory loss of the lateral upper arm. Typically presents 48 to 72 hours following surgery.
  - Treatment:
    - Self-limited; majority resolve within 6 months with no sequelae
  - Risk factors:
    - Excessive spinal cord drift
    - Ossified posterior longitudinal ligament
- **Postoperative neck pain and mobility loss:**
  - Incidence ranging from 40 to 60% and 20 to 50%, respectively
  - Unclear etiology; likely due to excessive stripping of paraspinal muscles from facet capsules and prolonged postoperative immobilization
  - Risk factors:
    - Intraoperative facet joint disruption

◼ Suggested Readings

1. Ratliff JK, Cooper PR. Cervical laminoplasty: a critical review. J Neurosurg 2003;98(3, Suppl):230–238
2. Gu Y, Cao P, Gao R, et al. Incidence and risk factors of C5 palsy following posterior cervical decompression: a systematic review. PLoS One 2014;9(8):e101933
3. Hosono N, Yonenobu K, Ono K. Neck and shoulder pain after laminoplasty. A noticeable complication. Spine 1996;21(17):1969–1973

6 Posterior Laminectomy and Fusion

Tips and Pearls before You Begin

A laminectomy accomplishes indirect decompression of the spinal cord by allowing posterior translation of the cord away from the anterior compressive pathology. In patients with **myeloradiculopathy** and significant radicular symptoms, the presence of foraminal stenosis should be identified on preoperative imaging studies and appropriate concomitant foraminotomies planned. During preoperative positioning, **excessive flexion or extension** should be avoided in myelopathic patients. For foraminotomies, slight flexion opens the interspaces and foramina, but care must be taken during dissection, as the dural sac is more susceptible to injury.

The surgical exposure for laminectomy proceeds caudal to cephalad; this facilitates subperiosteal detachment of paraspinal muscles, which attach in the same direction, and reduces bleeding. A clamp is placed on an exposed spinous process, and a lateral radiograph is obtained to confirm levels. Dissection should proceed to the lateral margin of the facet joints. This extent of exposure establishes the landmarks needed for safe placement of lateral mass screws and ensures that more than half of the facet joint is not removed during any associated foraminotomy. Dissection beyond the lateral margin of the facet joint risks significant bleeding from the soft-tissue musculature. Care must be taken to avoid injuring the facet capsules at any level if a fusion is not planned.

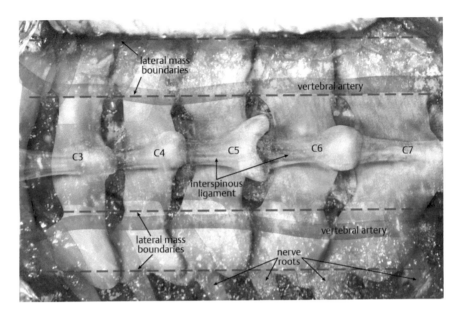

- A midline posterior approach is utilized, with the dissection performed through the avascular ligamentum nuchae.
- Subperiosteal exposure is performed, extending out to the lateral edge of the lateral mass:
  - Bleeding is typically encountered along the lateral edge of the lateral mass.
  - This bleeding can be controlled with bipolar cautery.

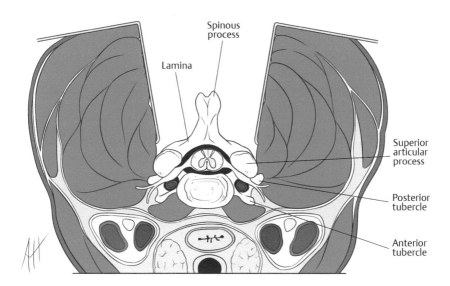

Cross section. Bilateral exposure of the posterior cervical spine with subperiosteal dissection of the paraspinal muscles. This approach is identical to that for the posterior cervical foraminotomy. The midline incision can be extended proximally toward the occiput to include as many levels as necessary. The approach is expanded laterally through dissection and retraction of the paracervical muscles beyond the facet joints until the transverse processes.

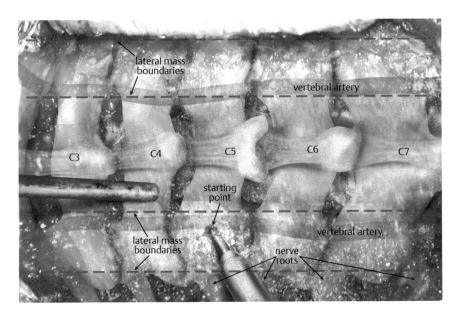

- The lateral mass is exposed and clearly defined, exposing the superior, inferior, and medial lateral borders.

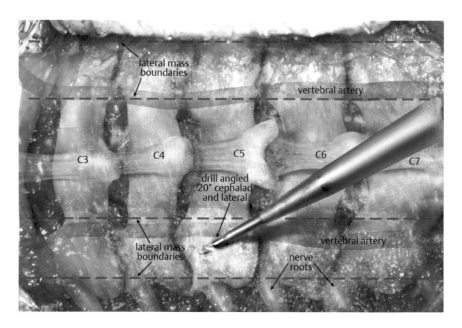

- Once the lateral mass is defined, the starting point should be created with a high-speed burr:
  - The center of the lateral mass is burred first.
  - The drill is then directed 20 degrees cephalad and lateral, thereby avoiding the vertebral artery and nerve root (Magerl's technique).

Potential Pitfalls

Vertebral artery injury can occur if drill placement is made directly anterior or 10 degrees medial to midpoint entry position.

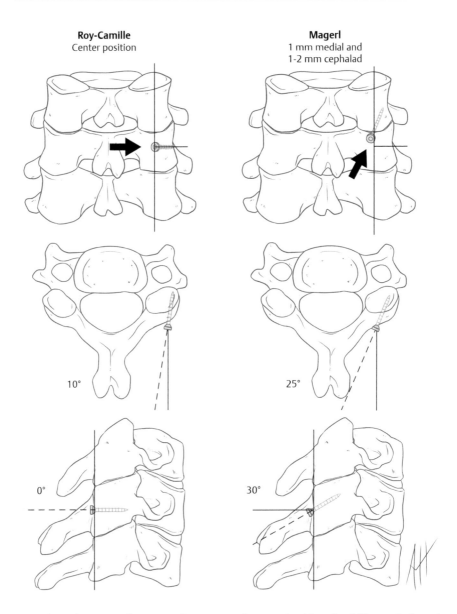

Magerl's and Roy-Camille's screw placement techniques. Position the drill superiorly and laterally to avoid the transverse foramen and concurrent arterial injury.

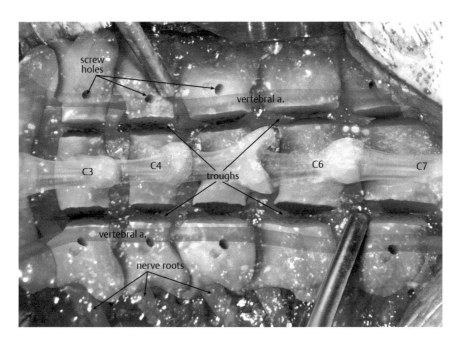

- Once the lateral mass screw holes are created, a laminectomy can be performed:
  - Two troughs are created with a high-speed burr.
  - The troughs are created just medial to the screw start points at the junction of the lateral mass and lamina.

Potential Pitfalls

Spinal cord injury can occur when utilizing Kerrison rongeurs for manual laminectomy.

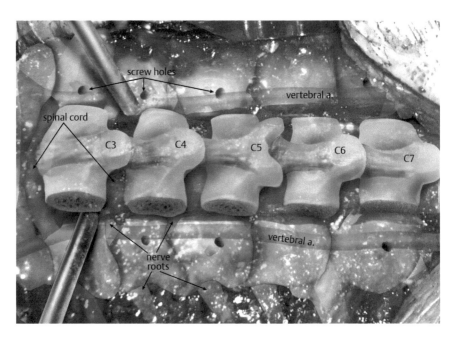

• The lamina is then removed en bloc with passage of instruments into the canal.

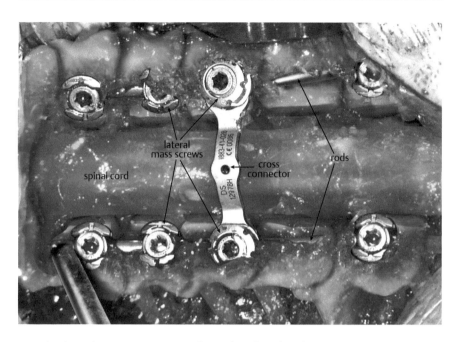

- The lateral mass screws are then placed and rods are secured in place. A cross-connector can be applied to increase torsional rigidity:
  - The bone graft is placed into the decorticated facet joints.

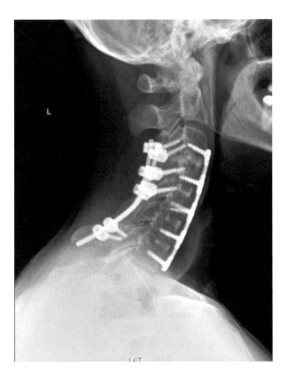

Postoperative radiographs. Seven-month postoperative visit of a patient with C3–C7 posterior cervical laminectomy and fusion with concomitant anterior diskectomy and fusion.

Perioperative Complications

- **Nerve root injury:**
  - Direct damage during foraminotomy or lateral screw placement.
  - Postsurgical C5 palsy most frequent (0.5–8% of patients):
    - Unknown etiology; likely due to posterior translation of spinal cord and subsequent stretching of the short C5 nerve root.
  - Prevention:
    - Maintain a cranial and lateral trajectory for lateral mass screws.
    - Avoid utilization of high-profile Kerrison rongeurs during foraminal decompression.
  - Treatment:
    - C5 palsy typically spontaneously resolves 6 to 12 months postoperatively.
- **Spinal cord injury and dural tears:**
  - Direct damage during laminectomy:
    - Manual laminectomies pose greatest risk from repetitive placement of instruments deep to the lamina.
  - Prevention:
    - Instrumentation with profiles larger than the footplate of a 2-mm Kerrison rongeur should not be placed near the central canal.
  - Treatment:
    - For dural tears and cerebrospinal fluid leaks, primary repair with nonabsorbable suture is preferred.
    - Head elevation to reduce pressure on the repair.
- **Postoperative epidural hematoma:**
  - Accumulation of postoperative edema and bleeding.
  - Characterized by gradual postoperative neurologic deficit.
  - Risk factors:
    - Increased number of levels.
    - History of coagulopathies or vascular anomalies.
  - Prevention:
    - Placement of subfascial surgical drain prior to surgical closure.
- **Vertebral artery injury:**
  - Damage from misdirected lateral mass screw.
  - Four to eight percent incidence during posterior cervical instrumented procedures.
  - Symptoms and treatment similar to vertebral artery injuries encountered during anterior cervical corpectomy and fusion.

◼ Suggested Readings

1. Awad JN, Kebaish KM, Donigan J, Cohen DB, Kostuik JP. Analysis of the risk factors for the development of post-operative spinal epidural haematoma. J Bone Joint Surg Br 2005;87(9):1248–1252
2. Schroeder GD, Hsu WK. Vertebral artery injuries in cervical spine surgery. Surg Neurol Int 2013;4(Suppl 5):S362–S367

7 Occipitocervical Fusion

For dual plating, occipital screws should be placed three to a side on either side of the midline, just below the superior nuchal line and as close to the external occipital protuberance as possible. An independent occipital plate may require only two or three screws, usually oriented in a vertical or transverse orientation. Leakage of cerebrospinal fluid (CSF) at this stage can usually be stopped by placing a screw or bone wax into the hole.

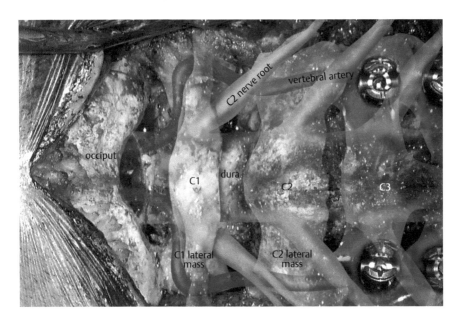

- A midline incision is made from the external occipital protuberance to the lowest level to be included in the fusion.
- Subperiosteal exposure of the occiput and the C1–C2 vertebral levels is essential for instrumentation placement.
- The vertebral artery travels along the superior lateral surface of the C1 arch approximately 1.5 cm from the midline.

Superficial landmarks include:

- External occipital protuberance:
  - Approximates the middle of the squamous portion of the occipital bone.
  - Most superior point is the inion.
- C2 spinous process.

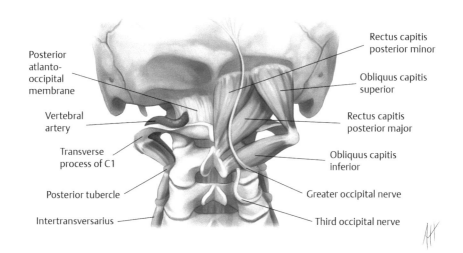

Posterior atlanto-occipital membrane

Rectus capitis posterior minor

Obliquus capitis superior

Vertebral artery

Rectus capitis posterior major

Transverse process of C1

Obliquus capitis inferior

Posterior tubercle

Greater occipital nerve

Intertransversarius

Third occipital nerve

Coronal section. The C2 nerve root is contained within the surgical field. The greater occipital nerve innervates the skin along the posterior aspect of the scalp.

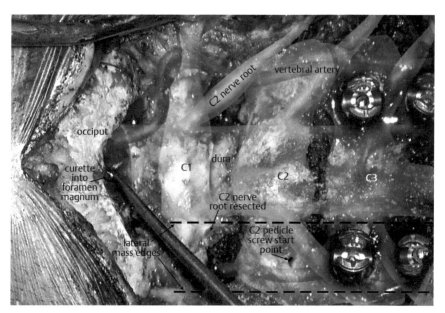

C2 nerve root

vertebral artery

occiput

curette into foramen magnum

C1

dura

C2

C3

C2 nerve root resected

lateral mass edges

C2 pedicle screw start point

- A curette is placed into the foramen magnum to clearly define the inferior border of the occiput.

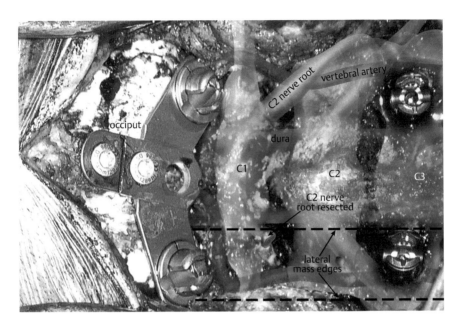

- An occipital plate has been applied. Screws are placed bicortically in the midline:
  - The plate is appropriately sized so that it is easier to connect the occipital and C1–C2 screw tulips.

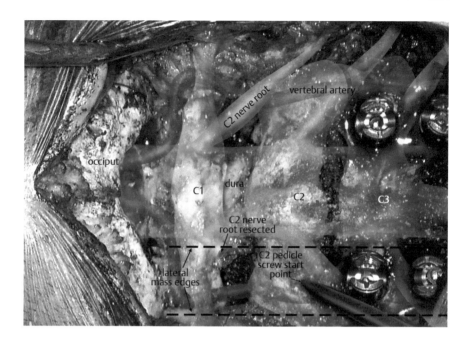

- The C2 (axis) pedicle screw starting point occurs at the inferior and lateral edge of the inferior articular process of C2:
  - The vertebral artery lies directly anterolateral. The screw should be directed medial and cephalad to avoid potential vascular injury.
    - Screws placed bicortically into the anterior axis may risk injury to the internal carotid artery:
      - The C2 screw is angled 20 degrees medially and 15 to 20 degrees caudally (use lateral fluoroscopy).

Potential Pitfalls

Vertebral artery injury can occur with excessive lateral and caudal screw placement. The artery passes from the transverse foramen of the atlas and then travels medially, piercing the lateral angle of the posterior atlanto-occipital membrane.

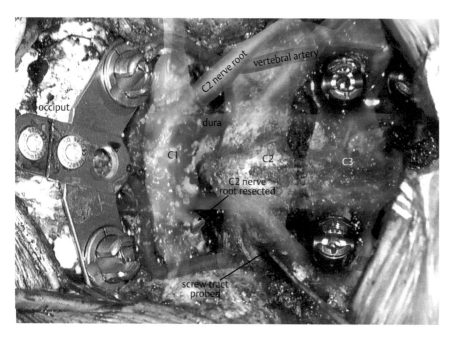

- The screw tract is drilled and then probed to ensure that the cortical walls are not breached.

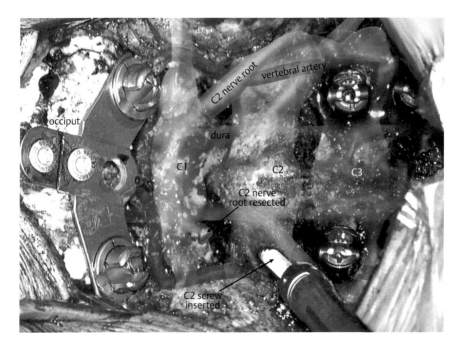

• The C2 pedicle screw is inserted.

Potential Pitfalls

A **narrow C2 pedicle** creates a high risk of breach into the neural canal. C2 translaminar screws can alternatively be used if concern for neural damage is high.

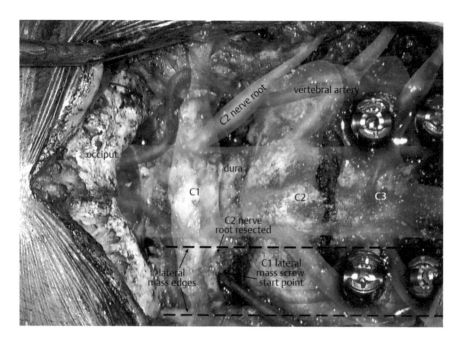

- The C1 (atlas) lateral mass screw starting point is inferior to the arch of C1. The C2 (occipital) nerve root has been resected to facilitate screw placement:
  - Resection of the C2 nerve may result in occipital dysesthesias in up to 20% of patients due to interruption of the greater occipital nerve.
- The ponticulus posticus (Latin for "little bridge to the rear") refers to a bony bridge on the atlas that covers the groove for the vertebral artery (also known as the arcuate foramen). It is a common anatomic variant that is estimated to occur in 3 to 15% of the population.

Potential Pitfalls

Damage to the extensive **C1–C2 venous plexus** can lead to significant hemorrhage. Bipolar coagulation or hemostatic agents can be used to control bleeding.

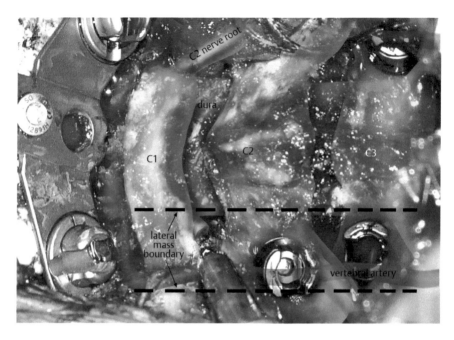

- C1 lateral mass screw placement is shown. Note that the C2 nerve root has been resected, exposing the C1 lateral mass and the C1–C2 facet joint.

Potential Pitfalls

Excessive advancement of the drill bit can lead to entry into the **retropharynx**. The drill should be stopped at the posterior aspect of the anterior C1 tubercle.

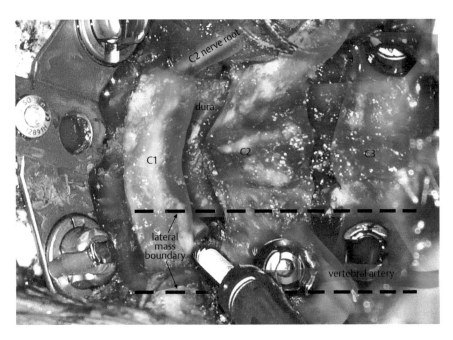

- The C1 screw tract is probed. A unicortical screw is placed. Bicortical screws are dangerous and may encroach upon the internal carotid artery anteriorly:
  - The C1 lateral mass screw is aimed 10 degrees medially and 10 degrees cranially (use lateral fluoroscopy).

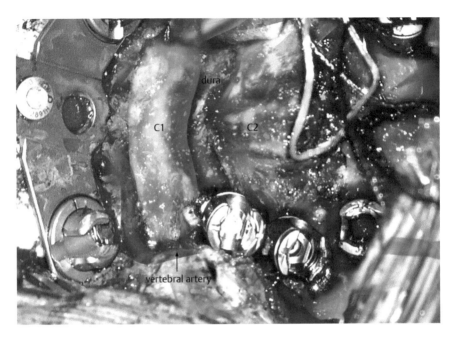

- The C1 lateral mass screw is inserted.

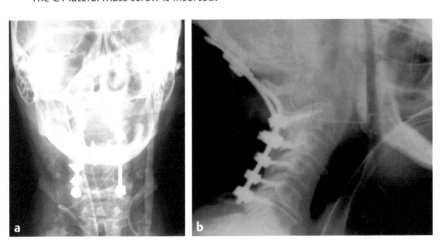

Postoperative radiographs. Postoperative **(a)** AP and **(b)** lateral radiographs (cervical spine) of a patient undergoing an occipito-cervical fusion (occiput and C2 screw fixation) for a C1-C2 leiomyosarcoma resection.

Perioperative Complications

- **Vertebral artery injury:**
  - Transection of the vertebral artery due to excessive lateral and/or caudad C2 screw placement.
  - Presents with hemorrhage and possible acute central nervous system ischemia.
  - Treatment:
    - Aggressive intravenous fluid resuscitation.
    - Placement of the head in a neutral position.
    - Hemostasis via digital pressure, Gelfoam.
    - Placement of the screw into the adjacent bone to tamponade bleeding.
    - Postoperative angiogram to evaluate for possible dissection.
  - Prevention:
    - Evaluation of arterial course on preoperative imaging.
- **Intraoperative dural tear, CSF leak, or neurologic injury:**
  - Occurs after placement of screws into the occiput or into a narrow C2 pedicle.
  - Characterized by orthostatic headache, nausea, vomiting.
  - Treatment:
    - Patch the defect with collagen matrix or tissue allograft.
    - Apply fibrin glue or sealant.
    - Consider lumbar drain to divert CSF.
  - Prevention:
    - Use of C2 translaminar screws can prevent dural or neurologic injury in cases of a narrow C2 pedicle.
- **Malpositioned occipital screws:**
  - Due to placement of screws in diseased bone (osteomyelitis, neoplasm)
  - Characterized by inadequate screw purchase
  - Prevention:
    - Place screws closer to the superior nuchal line, but no more than 20 mm lateral to the midline and as far superior to the foramen magnum as possible.
- **Pressure ulcers and bony erosion of the lamina:**
  - Caused by ill-fitting plates or rods.
  - Presents with pressure ulcers of the skin, erosion of the lamina, subsequent hardware exposure, and infection.
  - Treatment:
    - Revision procedure.
  - Prevention:
    - Verify a neutral occipitocervical alignment before locking in construct.

■ Suggested Readings

1.   Ahmed R, Menezes AH. Management of operative complications related to occipitocervical instrumentation. Neurosurgery 2013;72(2, Suppl Operative):ons214–ons228, discussion ons228

2.   He B, Yan L, Xu Z, Chang Z, Hao D. The causes and treatment strategies for the postoperative complications of occipitocervical fusion: a 316 cases retrospective analysis. Eur Spine J 2014;23(8):1720–1724

8 Thoracic Pedicle Screw Placement

■ Posterior Thoracic/Lumbar

- Posterior spinal fusions
- Scoliosis correction
- Removal of tumors of the posterior vertebral body
- Stabilization of vertebral fractures via vertebroplasty/kyphoplasty
- Open biopsy

■ Positioning

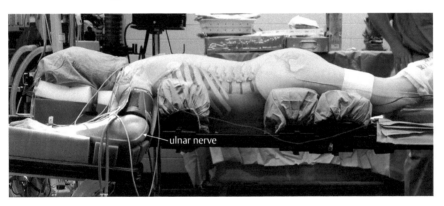

ulnar nerve

For cases that involve a posterior thoracic and lumbar procedure, the Jackson table is often preferred. The Jackson table is radiolucent and allows for the chest and hip pads to be placed independently. The chest pads should be placed at the level of the manubrium and below the axilla. The hip pads should be placed just below the anterior superior iliac spine. The thigh pads are often placed immediately below the hip pad. When the chest and thigh pads are placed this way, it allows the abdomen to hang freely, increasing lumbar lordosis and decreasing venous bleeding during the surgical procedure. The neck is placed into a neutral position, with care being taken to protect the eyes from pressure.

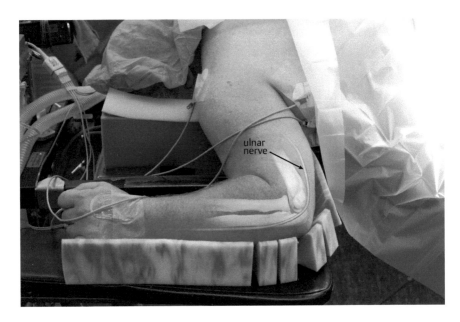

The arms are placed into a 90–90 position, with a foam pad placed to prevent compression along the ulnar nerve. The shoulder should not be hyperextended, thereby decreasing the likelihood of rotator cuff impingement.

Superficial landmarks include:

- Gluteal cleft
- C7–T1 spinous processes:
  – Largest spinous processes in the surgical region

Tips and Pearls before You Begin

Meticulous dissection with exposure of the transverse processes is mandatory. Facetectomies should be performed at each fusion level, and the cartilage should be removed. Fluoroscopy or intraoperative radiographs can be used to identify the pedicle shadow. The most important anatomic landmark is the middle of the facet, as the pedicle screw start point should always be lateral to this midpoint.

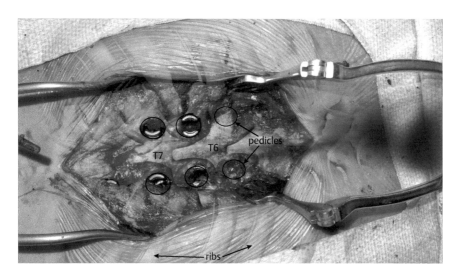

Meticulous dissection should be performed with the inferior 3 to 5 mm of the inferior facet osteotomized. The base of the superior articular process is a key landmark for entry into the pedicle. The starting point for each thoracic screw varies. Biomechanically, it is best to place the screws parallel to the superior end plate. When the procedure is started distal at T12, there is a trend toward a more medial and cephalad pedicle starting point as one proceeds toward the midthoracic region (T7–T8). Proximal to this point, the starting point moves more lateral and caudad as one proceeds to the upper thoracic spine.

Internervous Plane

The paraspinal muscles are innervated by the posterior rami of the individual nerve roots. As these nerves do not cross the midline, a midline incision will be in the internervous plane.

Potential Pitfalls

Segmental vessels coming off the aorta supply the paraspinal muscles and appear between the transverse processes. Cauterization of these vessels is necessary to prevent excessive bleeding.

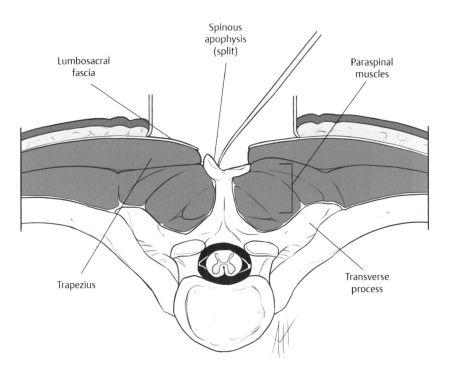

Cross section. Superficial and deep exposure. Paraspinal muscles split and retracted laterally. To widen the exposure, self-retaining retractors can be used and the dissection can be carried out to the tips of the transverse processes.

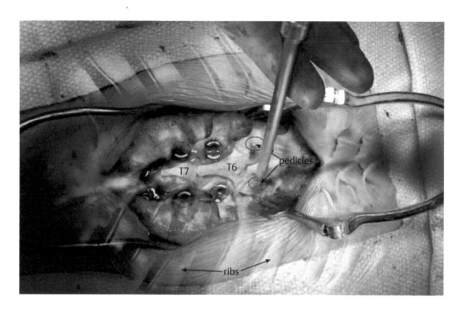

- A burr may be used to create a pedicle blush by removing only the dorsal cortex in the area of the targeted pedicle entry point.

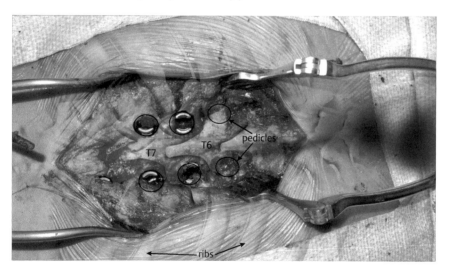

- Pedicle blush refers to bleeding that arises from the vertebral body into the pedicle start point.

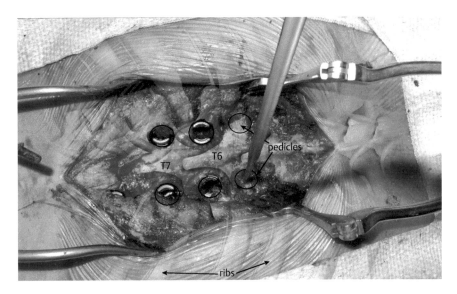

- With gentle but firm ventral pressure, the gear shift should be easily wiggled into the pedicle. If any amount of significant resistance is met, the surgeon should reevaluate the starting point and trajectory of the pedicle. The gear shift should be advanced approximately 30 to 35 mm.

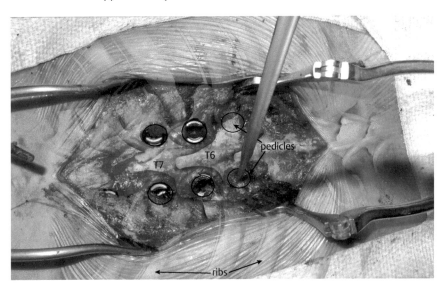

- The surgeon then probes the pedicle hole in order to palpate the medial, lateral, superior, inferior, and ventral walls of the pedicle. Most pedicle violations occur at the junction of the pedicle and vertebral body (15–20 mm depth).

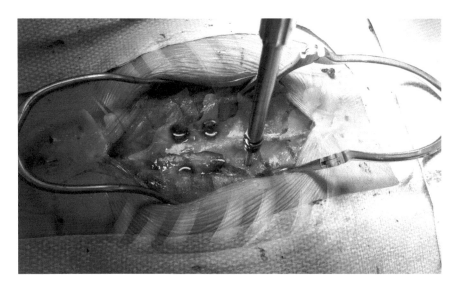

- The screw is then approximately sized and positioned. Typical screw lengths in the lower thoracic spine average 40 to 45 mm, while in the upper thoracic spine lengths may be as short as 35 mm.

Potential Pitfalls

Pedicle violation can occur with excess screw length or malpositioning. Violations commonly occur in the anterior, medial, lateral, and inferior aspects of the pedicle.

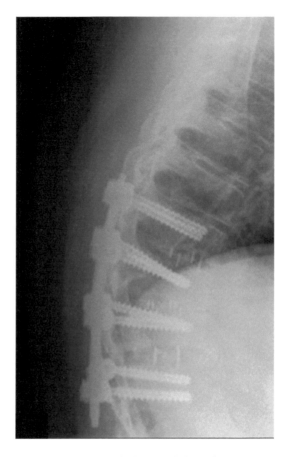

Sagittal view. Postoperative radiograph showing bilateral pedicle screw placement in multiple levels throughout the thoracolumbar spine.

Perioperative Complications

- Pedicle violation:
  - Caused by malpositioning of screws in the anterior, medial, lateral, or inferior direction.
  - Presents with:
    - Nerve root or spinal cord injury (inferior or medial violation).
    - Injuries to the aorta, segmental vessels, lung parenchyma, pneumothorax (lateral/ventral violation).
    - Injuries to the aorta, vena cava, esophagus (ventral violation).
  - Prevention:
    - Screw placement confirmation with intraoperative anteroposterior and lateral radiographs, fluoroscopy, or computed tomography (CT) scan.
    - Postoperative CT scan can confirm placement of the screws and integrity of nearby visceral and neurovascular structures.
- Screw pullout/failure of fixation:
  - Caused by malpositioned pedicle screws, poor screw purchase, or inadequate bone stock.
  - Prevention:
    - Use of screw augmentation via polymethylmethacrylate, hydroxyapatite, calcium phosphate, or carbonated apatite in at-risk patient.

■ Suggested Readings

1. Nimjee SM, Karikari IO, Carolyn A Hardin AB, et al. Safe and accurate placement of thoracic and thoracolumbar percutaneous pedicle screws without image-navigation. Asian J Neurosurg 2015;10(4):272–275
2. Bydon M, Xu R, Amin AG, et al. Safety and efficacy of pedicle screw placement using intraoperative computed tomography: consecutive series of 1148 pedicle screws. J Neurosurg Spine 2014;21(3):320–328
3. Gautschi OP, Schatlo B, Schaller K, Tessitore E. Clinically relevant complications related to pedicle screw placement in thoracolumbar surgery and their management: a literature review of 35,630 pedicle screws. Neurosurg Focus 2011;31(4):E8

9 Minimally Invasive Thoracic Corpectomy

■ Lateral/Thoracic/Lumbar Positioning

- Abscess drainage
- Vertebral body biopsy and resection
- Anterolateral spinal decompression
- Anterior spinal fusion

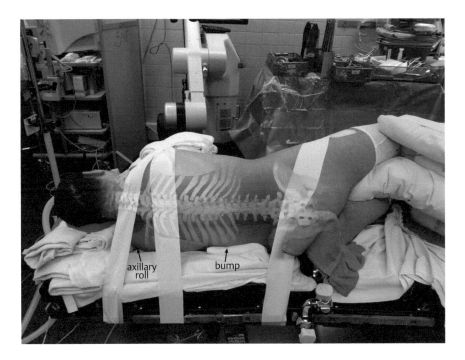

The patient is positioned on a regular operating room table with a bump underneath the affected level. The patient is also positioned with the operative site over the break in the bed, allowing the patient to be maximally flexed at the surgical level (if necessary).

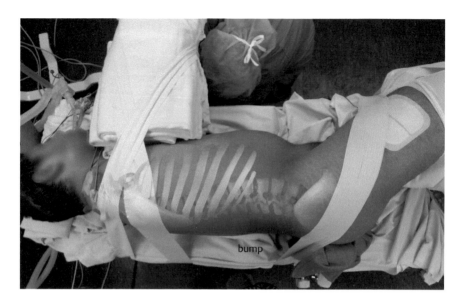

Tape is used to secure the pelvis and the thorax such that flexion can be accomplished without movement of the patient on the operating table. The arms are well padded, and an axillary roll should be placed under the patient to avoid any brachial plexopathies.

Superficial landmarks include:

- Ribs and associated intercostal space adjacent to the desired level.
- Spinous processes of the levels of interest:
  - Confirmation via fluoroscopy is necessary.

Tips and Pearls before You Begin

Care should be taken to obtain orthogonal fluoroscopic views of the involved vertebral level. Parallax may result in exposure of the incorrect vertebral body and improper dilator placement along the anterior vertebral body, risking damage to the great vessels. Blunt dissection is necessary to prevent perforation of the pleura. A sponge stick or peanut can be used to sweep the pleura anteriorly. If the pleura is violated, then a chest tube or red rubber catheter can be placed upon completion of surgery. In general, most patients are asymptomatic, and prompt removal of the catheter will allow rapid mobilization.

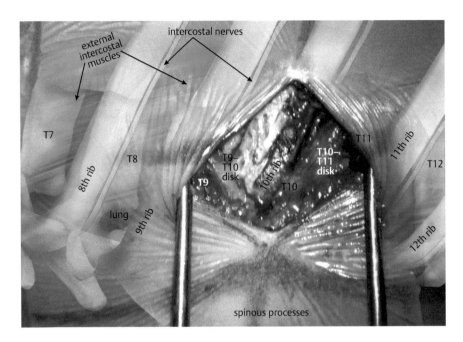

Rib exposure. The anterior and posterior margins of the vertebral body to be resected are marked under fluoroscopy. The overlying rib is subperiosteally exposed.

Internervous Plane

There is no internervous plane in this approach. The muscles of the abdominal wall, which are divided in line with the skin incision, are segmentally innervated. No significant denervation occurs.

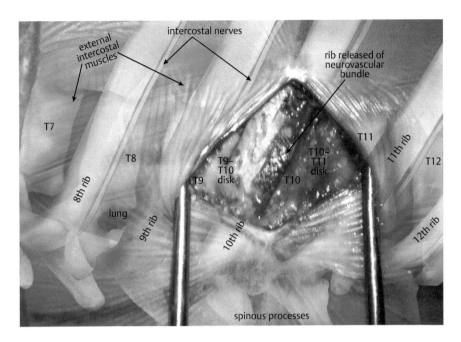

- The inferior portion of the rib is subperiosteally released from the neurovascular bundle.

Potential Pitfalls

Hemorrhage of the **segmental intercostal arteries** often occurs during rib exposure. Hemostasis can be obtained via ligation or cauterization. Understanding that the neurovascular bundle lies at the inferior edge of the rib will help expedite hemostasis.

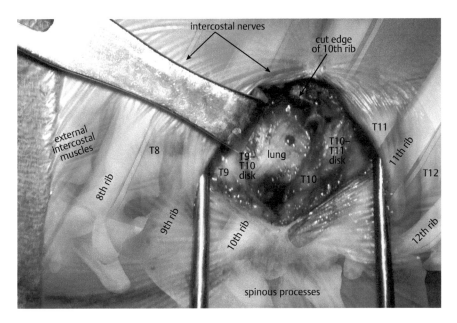

intercostal nerves

cut edge
of 10th rib

external
intercostal
muscles

T8

T11

T10–
T11
disk

T9–
T10
disk   lung

T9   T10

T12

8th rib

9th rib

10th rib

11th rib

12th rib

spinous processes

- Approximately 2 cm of rib have been resected. The pleura of the lung is visualized.

Potential Pitfalls

Pleural violation can occur during subperiosteal resection of the rib. If a pneumothorax occurs, the placement of a catheter or chest tube may be necessary.

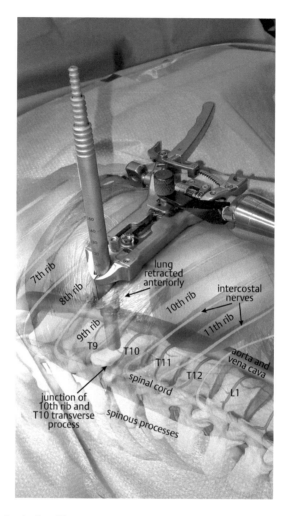

- A series of tubular dilators are placed into the defect, sweeping the lung and pleura anteriorly and resulting in an extrapleural exposure of the vertebral body.

Potential Pitfalls

Migration or misplacement of the tubular dilators can lead to disorientation in relation to anatomical landmarks.

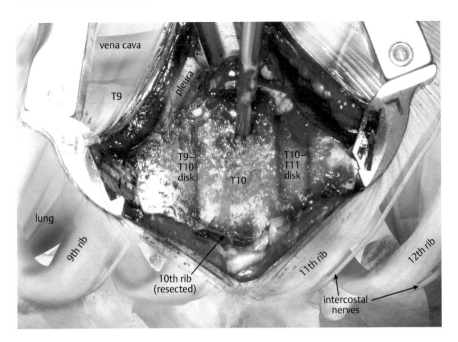

- The intervertebral disk space above and below the involved vertebral level is subperiosteally exposed. The segmental artery has been cauterized and resected.

Potential Pitfalls

Retraction of the **thoracic spinal cord** can lead to permanent neurologic deficits. Resection of additional lateral bone and tissue can improve dilator angulation and exposure.

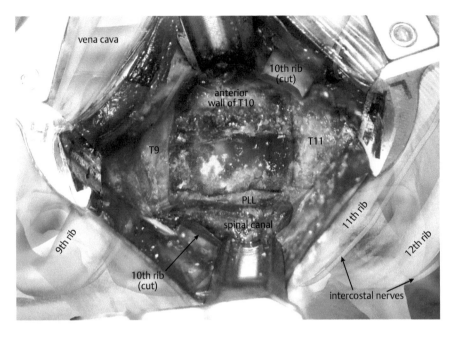

- The corpectomy has been completed using a high-speed burr. The anterior vertebral body wall has been thinned and preserved, while the T9–T10 and T10–T11 disk spaces have been resected. The spinal canal has been exposed, preserving the posterior longitudinal ligament.

Potential Pitfalls

Resection of the **anterior vertebral body wall** can lead to compromise of the ventral neurovascular structures.

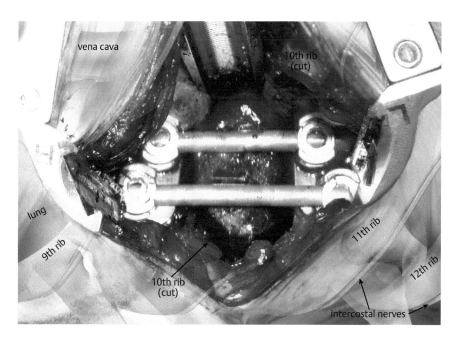

- An expandable titanium cage has been appropriately sized and placed into the defect. A plate has been placed into the vertebral body above and below at the T9 and T11 levels, respectively.

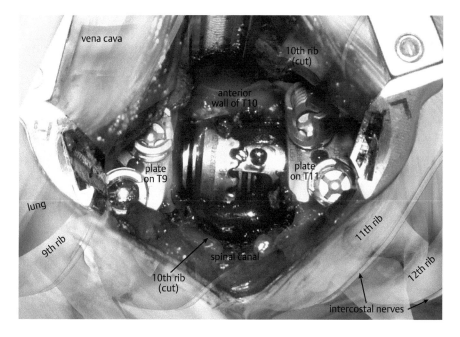

- A dual-rod construct has secured the T9 and T11 levels.

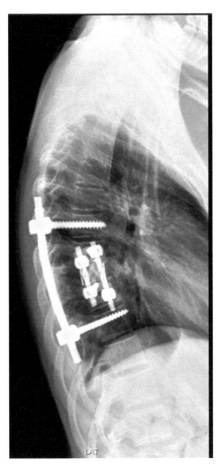

Sagittal view. Postoperative radiograph demonstrating T8 corpectomy with expandable cage and dual-rod construct.

Perioperative Complications

- **Pleural violation:**
  - Occurs during subperiosteal resection of the rib and associated fascia.
  - Presents with possible pneumothorax and respiratory insufficiency.
  - Prevention:
    - Gentle and meticulous subperiosteal resection.
  - Treatment:
    - Catheterization or placement of a chest tube if the patient is symptomatic.
- **Neurologic injury—durotomy, cerebrospinal fluid (CSF) leakage, neurologic deficit:**
  - Occurs with retraction of the thoracic spinal cord or during resection of the vertebral body.
  - Presents with orthostatic headache, nausea, vomiting, focal neurologic deficits.
  - Prevention:
    - Avoidance of thoracic spinal cord retraction.
    - Resection of bone and tissue laterally to allow for medial angulation of tubular dilators and improved exposure.
  - Treatment:
    - Placement of a water-insoluble layer and dural sealant in cases of durotomy.
    - Possible lumbar CSF drain.
- **Arterial injury:**
  - Due to improper docking of the dilator too far anteriorly or resection of the anterior vertebral body wall.
  - Presents with hemorrhage and possible acute central nervous system ischemia.
  - Prevention:
    - Avoid removal of anterior vertebral body wall.
  - Treatment:
    - Cauterization of the bleeding segmental vessel(s).
    - Stop the procedure and provide vigorous intraoperative fluid resuscitation and hemostasis with hemostatic agents and pressure.
    - Immediate vascular surgery consultation for management guidance.

Suggested Readings

1. Lall RR, Smith ZA, Wong AP, Miller D, Fessler RG. Minimally invasive thoracic corpectomy: surgical strategies for malignancy, trauma, and complex spinal pathologies. Minim Invasive Surg 2012;2012:213791
2. Kasliwal MK, Deutsch H. Minimally invasive retropleural approach for central thoracic disc herniation. Minim Invasive Neurosurg 2011;54(4):167–171

10 Percutaneous Vertebral Cement Augmentation

The use of **biplanar fluoroscopy** greatly aids in cannula insertion and cement injection. The lateral image is brought over the top or under the bed, with the arc leaning away toward the head. The anteroposterior (AP) image is brought in diagonally, with the image intensifier directly over the target site. It is most convenient to obtain the true AP image first, because the diagonal entry makes this process challenging. The lateral image is then adjusted to accommodate the AP image.

Treatment of multiple levels can be performed with a single batch of cement. The cement is stored in a sterile ice water bath to slow the polymerization process. With **vertebroplasty**, all the cannulas are inserted first, and then each site is injected sequentially. With **kyphoplasty**, the first site is drilled, the balloon tamp deployed, and the cement injected. The limit on the number of levels is dictated by the cement load. The risk of **cement toxicity** increases with the number of levels treated. As a general rule, no more than three levels are treated in one operation.

Special consideration related to cement fill is needed for **kyphoplasty**. Along with the cement required for filling the void created by the balloon tamp, additional cement is needed to allow the integration of the cement into the surrounding trabecular bone. This serves to lock in the cement. Inadequate filling may lead to further **collapse** of the surrounding bone from excessive motion at the interface between the bone and cement. In general, the volume of cement injected should be greater than the volume of the inflated balloon.

Maintenance of the reduction via **kyphoplasty** may be difficult in certain fractures, particularly in vertebrae plana. Once the balloon is deflated, the fracture may collapse again. The restoration of vertebral body height can be maintained by the eggshell technique. A small amount of cement (0.5 to 1 mL) is injected into the cavity. The balloon tamp is reinserted and gently re-elevated. The small cement bolus is then spread around the balloon to create a thin eggshell of cement. When the balloon is removed, the eggshell mantle holds the reduction until the remainder of the cement is injected.

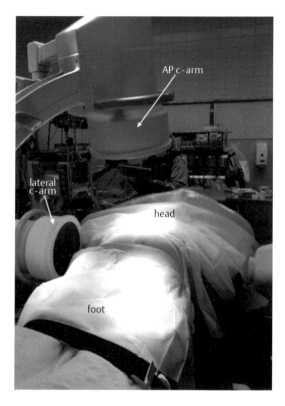

• Biplanar fluoroscopy is used throughout the procedure.

• Thoracic spinous processes:
  – Fluoroscopic confirmation of the affected level is required.

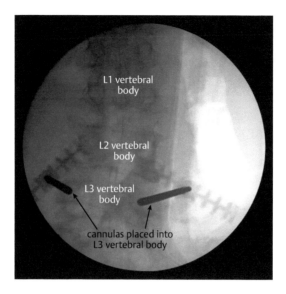

- The starting position for the cannula should be at the 10 o'clock or 2 o'clock position of the pedicle (superior-lateral corner depending on the left or right side of the spine). This position places the cannula the farthest from the exiting nerve root. The cannula is advanced such that on the AP side it never crosses the medial edge of the pedicle until it crosses the posterior vertebral body line on the lateral image.

Potential Pitfalls

Fluoroscopic visualization can be hindered by disease processes such as osteoporosis. Position of the C-arms may require adjustment to obtain adequate images in those cases.

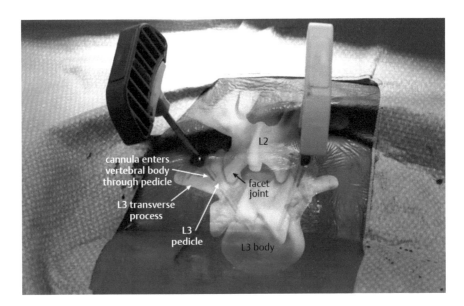

- The cannula is started lateral to the facet joint, thereby avoiding any damage to the facet capsule.

Potential Pitfalls

Hemothorax, pneumothorax, and soft-tissue hematomas can result from improper instrument positioning. Adequate visualization of instruments on imaging is necessary in prevention of these complications.

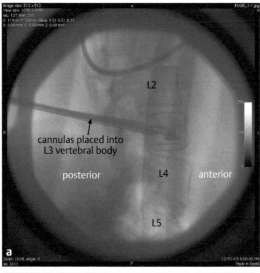

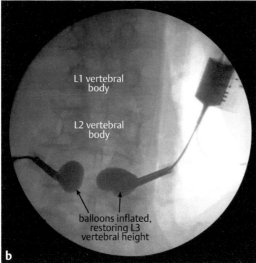

- Fluoroscopy is used to confirm that the balloon is in the anterior portion of the vertebral body, so that no bone can be retropulsed into the spinal canal.

Potential Pitfalls

Neurological injury and decline can occur with improper balloon placement in the posterior vertebral body. Retropulsion of posterior bone fragments can lead to spinal cord injury.

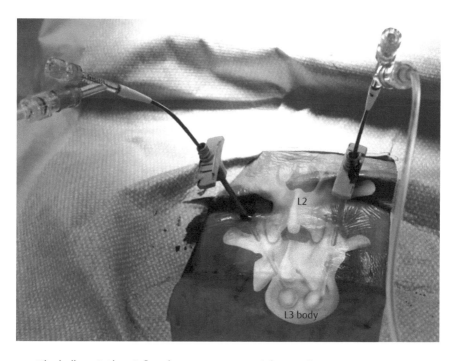

- The balloon is then inflated to create a potential space for cement augmentation.

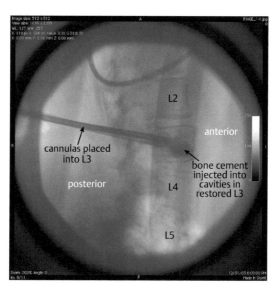

- Cement is then added to the vertebral body under fluoroscopic visualization. The cement is carefully observed on both the AP and lateral images so that the borders of the vertebral body are not violated. If cement extravasation is noted, the procedure is terminated. Cement should be avoided in the posterior aspect of the vertebral body.

Potential Pitfalls

Cement leakage can occur, resulting from fracture clefts or improper instrument positioning. Prevention involves use of adequate imaging, slow injection of cement material, and improving visualization of cement with the addition of barium.

Perioperative Complications

- **Cement embolization to pulmonary vasculature:**
  - Occurs via leakage of bone cement into the draining vertebral venous plexus.
  - Presents with tachypnea, tachycardia, chest pain, hemoptysis.
  - Management:
    - Obtain computed tomography (CT) scan to evaluate for pulmonary embolism.
    - Definitive treatment based on symptomatology:
      - Asymptomatic—observation of clinical progress.
      - Symptomatic—anticoagulation with or without surgical removal of embolus.
  - Prevention:
    - Proper fluoroscopic visualization of vertebral body and cement.
    - Slow administration of cement.
- **Cement leakage:**
  - Caused by fracture clefts or improper instrument positioning.
  - Presents with neurologic deficits if leakage occurs into the spinal canal; adjacent vertebral fracture occurs if leakage involves the associated disk space.
  - Prevention:
    - Adequate fluoroscopic visualization with slow injection.
    - Addition of barium to the cement for easier visualization.
- **Pedicle fracture:**
  - Caused by improper cannula insertion.
  - Presents with back pain, possible neurologic deficits if there is spinal cord/nerve root involvement.
  - Prevention:
    - Placement of the cannula starting point at the superolateral border of the pedicle.
  - Management:
    - Nondisplaced, isolated fractures can be treated nonoperatively.
    - Displaced fractures with neurologic deficits require surgical reduction and fixation.

Perioperative Complications *(continued)*

- **Neurologic injury:**
  - Caused by inflation of the balloon in the posterior aspect of the vertebral body, leads to retropulsion of bone fragments.
  - Presents with focal neurologic deficits, radiculopathy, myelopathy.
  - Prevention:
    - Adequate fluoroscopic visualization to determine balloon placement prior to inflation.
- **Hemothorax, pneumothorax, soft-tissue hematomas:**
  - Caused by improper instrument positioning.
  - Management:
    - Catheter or drain placement for evacuation.
  - Prevention:
    - Adequate visualization of instruments on imaging.
- **Inadequate cement fill:**
  - Prevention:
    - Adequate fluoroscopic visualization to determine quantity of cement injected.

■ Suggested Readings

1. Awad BI, Lubelski D, Carmody M, et al. Surgical versus nonsurgical treatment of subaxial cervical pedicle fractures. World Neurosurg 2014;82(5):855–865
2. Krueger A, Bliemel C, Zettl R, Ruchholtz S. Management of pulmonary cement embolism after percutaneous vertebroplasty and kyphoplasty: a systematic review of the literature. Eur Spine J 2009;18(9):1257–1265
3. Truumees E, Hilibrand A, Vaccaro AR. Percutaneous vertebral augmentation. Spine J 2004;4(2):218–229
4. Yimin Y, Zhiwei R, Wei M, Jha R. Current status of percutaneous vertebroplasty and percutaneous kyphoplasty--a review. Med Sci Monit 2013;19:826–836

11 Open Laminectomy and Diskectomy

■ Posterior Lumbar Positioning

Indications for Posterior Lumbar Positioning:

- Removal of lumbar disk herniations.
- Decompression of nerve roots.
- Placement of posterior instrumentation.

Positioning of posterior lumbar procedures is similar to that of posterior thoracic procedures. Please refer to **Chapter 8: Thoracic Pedicle Screw Placement** *for detailed positioning instructions.*

Superficial landmarks include:

- Iliac crest:
    - Highest level typically lies at the L4–L5 intervertebral space.
- Spinous processes[a]:
    - The lumbar spinous processes are easily palpable.
- [a] Note: Ideal method of identifying target level is to insert a needle into the spinous process and obtain a radiograph.

Tips and Pearls before You Begin

The **ligamentum flavum** is often hypertrophied as part of the pathologic process. In the hypertrophied state, it can become a visual barrier to precise identification of neurological structures and may pose a physical impediment to safe entry into the **spinal canal**. To obviate these problems, excise the **superficial layers of the ligamentum** separately. A plane of dissection can be found at the lower attachment of the ligamentum to the top surface of the inferior lamina. The primary connection of the **ligamentum** is fixed to the leading surface of the **inferior lamina**. A hypertrophied ligamentum will generally expand posteriorly and mushroom up over the posterior, flat face of the lamina. Careful dissection with a small 2–0 or 3–0 curette, with the blunt aspect against the flat of the inferior lamina, usually defines the superficial layer for removal. The remaining **deep ligamentum** can then be excised. Always release the attachment of the deep layer from the undersurface of the superior lamina first (with the ligamentum still under tension). A small curette is used to sweep under the lamina. This minimizes the risk of **dural tear**. Releasing the inferior attachment first would slacken the ligament and require blind grasping under the superior lamina to remove the upper ligamentum. Blind use of a rongeur increases the risk of dural tears.

If the interlaminar space requires enlargement, this is best done with a side-cutting burr. To prevent **dural compromise**, keep the angle of the burr perpendicular to the dura so the noncutting tip is adjacent to vital structures. A horizontal sweeping motion is used, and care is taken to avoid downward pressure. Take care to preserve the pars interarticularis (7–9 mm minimum).

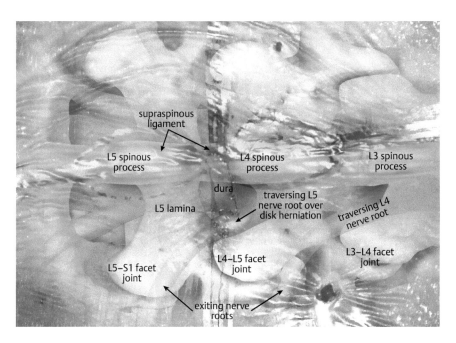

• A midline incision is used over the levels that are to be resected.

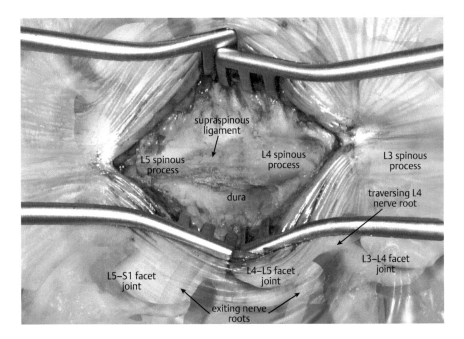

- The fascia is clearly identified prior to incision.

Internervous Plane

No internervous plane is present during this superficial dissection. The platysma muscle directly beneath the fascial sheath will be incised with the skin. It is innervated by branches of the facial nerve superiorly.

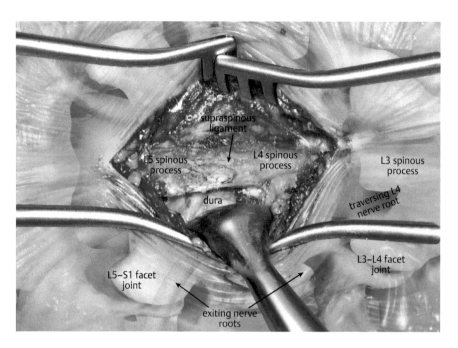

- The fascia is then opened in the midline over the spinous process. Subperiosteal dissection is accomplished with a Cobb elevator.

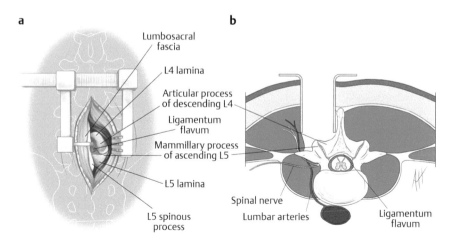

(a) *Top-down view and* **(b)** *cross-sectional view.* Paraspinal muscles are dissected subperiosteally and retracted laterally to adequately expose the laminae. Note the penetrating branches of the lumbar arteries.

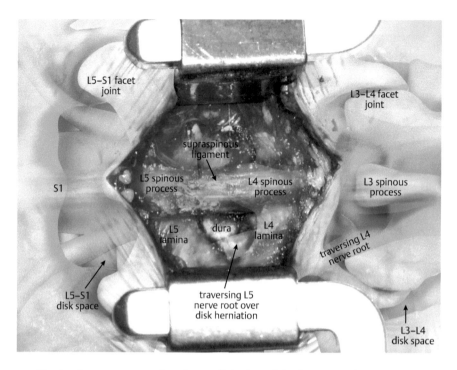

• The laminae are exposed to the medial edge of the facet capsule.

Potential Pitfalls

The **paraspinal vessels** run segmentally near the facet joints. During lateral dissection, these vessels can cause a moderate amount of bleeding; cauterization may be utilized to eliminate excessive bleeding.

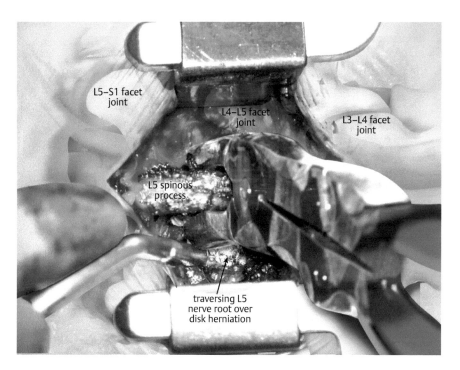

- The inferior half of the L4 and the superior half of the L5 spinous processes are removed along with the supraspinous and interspinous ligaments.

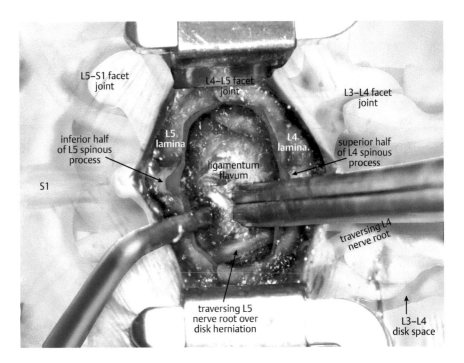

- A Kerrison rongeur is used to remove the ligamentum flavum.

Potential Pitfalls

A **hypertrophied ligamentum flavum** can prevent proper identification of nearby structures. Avoid blind resection of ligamentum to reduce the risk of **dural tears**.

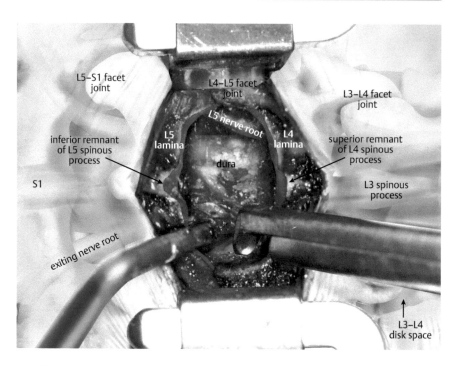

- The lateral recess is decompressed by undercutting the superior articular process of the inferior vertebrae.

Potential Pitfalls

Iatrogenic fractures can occur from excessive removal of the **pars interarticularis** and the **inferior articular process**. Avoid unnecessary thinning of these structures to prevent fractures or instability.

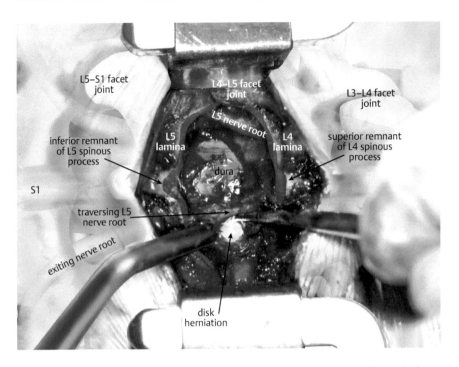

- The traversing nerve root is gently retracted medially, exposing the underlying disk herniation. The dura and the traversing nerve root are exposed.

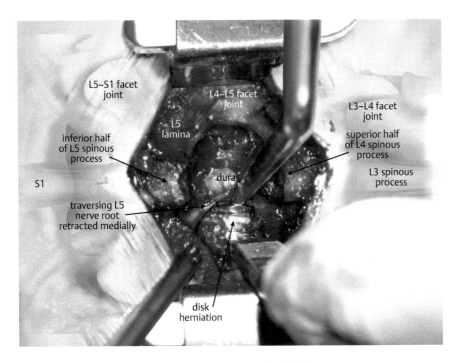

- A knife is used to make an annulotomy over the disk herniation.

Potential Pitfalls

Diskectomies have previously been performed at the **incorrect level**, often-times at the level above the intended target. If the expected pathology is not found, additional confirmatory imaging should be performed to establish the appropriate levels prior to incising the annulus.

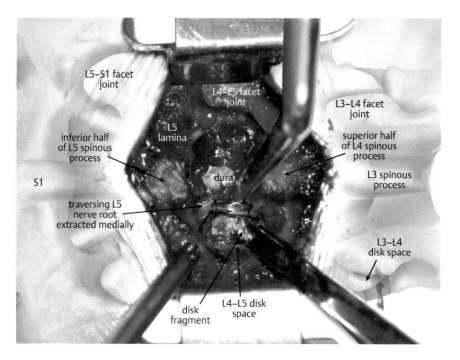

- The disk fragment is removed with a pituitary rongeur.

Potential Pitfalls

Injury to the iliac vessels can occur during disk removal if the rongeur breaches the **anterior longitudinal ligament** (ALL). Proper understanding of ALL location is necessary to avoid penetration of retroperitoneal vessels.

Perioperative Complications

- **Cerebrospinal fluid leak:**
  - Dural tear during ligamentum flavum resection or excessive retraction of dura:
    - Incidence of 5 to 8%.
  - Prevention:
    - Increase exposure size to avoid excessive nerve traction during herniation excision.
    - Initial removal of superficial layer of pathologic ligamentum flavum, with release and removal of the deep ligamentum afterward.
- **Intraoperative bleeding:**
  - Rupture of thin-walled epidural vessels surrounding the nerve roots and vertebrae during blunt dissection in the spinal canal.
  - Treatment:
    - Control bleeding with hemostatic sponges (such as Gelfoam or bipolar cautery).
    - Placement of wound drains usually not routinely necessary.
- **Vascular injury:**
  - Damage to the iliac vessels due to penetration of the ALL during disk removal.
  - Characterized by sudden hemorrhaging from disk space or abrupt hypotension.
  - Treatment:
    - Immediate wound closure
    - Reposition the patient to supine
    - Aggressive intravenous fluid resuscitation
    - Vascular surgery consult
- **Iatrogenic fractures or instability:**
  - Excessive thinning of the pars interarticularis or inferior articular process during laminectomy.
  - Prevention:
    - Minimize cutting or drilling of medial facet joint; avoid drilling of pars:
      ○ No more than one-third of medial facet should be removed.

Suggested Readings

1. Caputy AJ, Luessenhop AJ. Long-term evaluation of decompressive surgery for degenerative lumbar stenosis. J Neurosurg 1992;77(5):669–676 PubMed
2. German JW, Adamo MA, Hoppenot RG, Blossom JH, Nagle HA. Perioperative results following lumbar discectomy: comparison of minimally invasive discectomy and standard microdiscectomy. Neurosurg Focus 2008;25(2):E20 PubMed

12 Open Posterolateral Lumbar Fusion

Tips and Pearls before You Begin

In the lumbar spine, the **pedicles** are medially oriented, particularly in the lower lumbar segments. A lateral fluoroscopic image obtained for purposes of localization is extremely helpful in determining cephalad/caudad orientation of the pedicle. In general, the **L3 pedicle** is directed straight vertically toward the floor, with the upper lumbar segments angulated toward the head and the lower lumbar levels directed toward the foot. If a pedicle cannot be cannulated, a **hemilaminotomy** can be performed, palpating the medial wall to determine angulation.

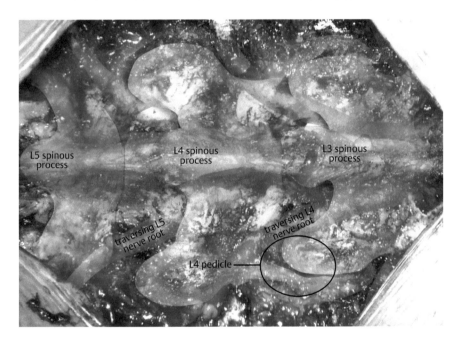

- The initial exposure should involve subperiosteal dissection of the muscles to the facet joint.

Internervous Plane

As encountered in the open lumbar laminectomy and diskectomy procedure, the **paraspinal vessels** run segmentally near the facet joints. During lateral dissection, these vessels can cause a moderate amount of bleeding; cauterization may be utilized to eliminate excessive bleeding.

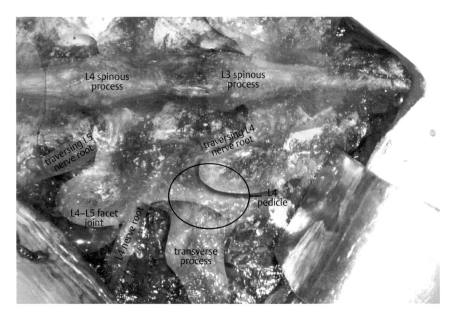

- Resection of the facet capsule and exposure of the superior articular process (caudad vertebra) and the transverse process are essential to identify the starting point for the lumbar pedicle screw.

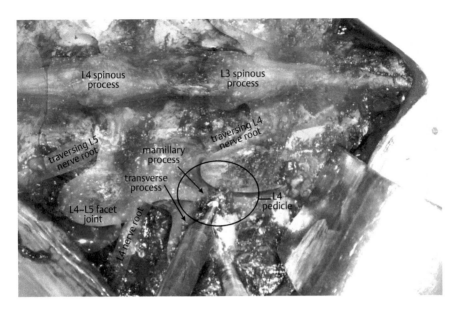

- Pedicle start point. The transverse process is bisected, and the mamillary process is identified at the junction of the inferolateral corner of the facet joint.

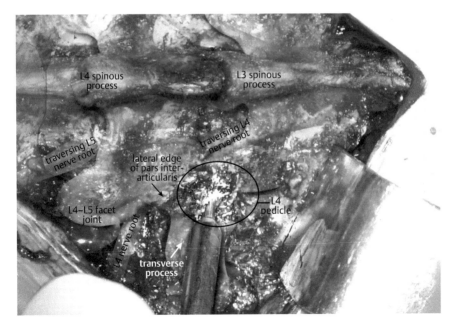

- The pars interarticularis is used to identify the medial extent of the pedicle.

a

b

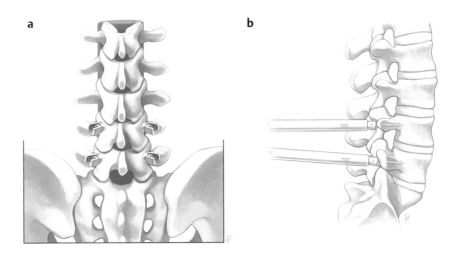

Anteroposterior (a) and lateral (b) views. Entry point is located on the lateral pars interarticularis, inferior to the facet joint at the level of the bisected transverse process. Note the changing positions of pedicle screw placement as one traverses caudally.

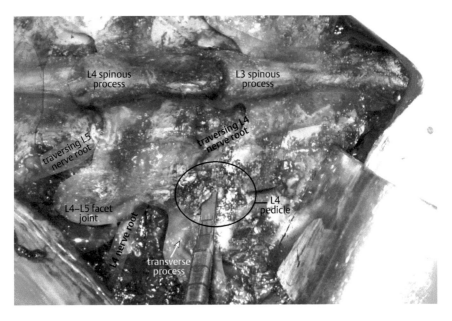

- The gear shift is advanced with gentle pressure and slight medial angulation.

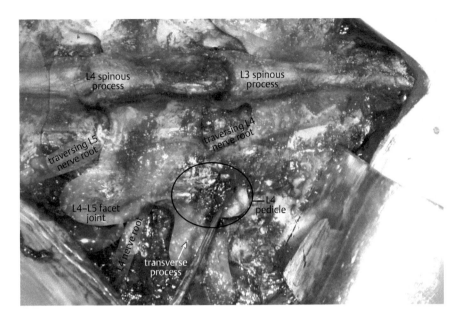

- The four walls of the pedicle are probed.

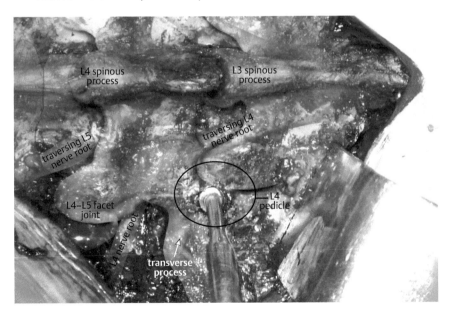

- The pedicle tract is tapped.

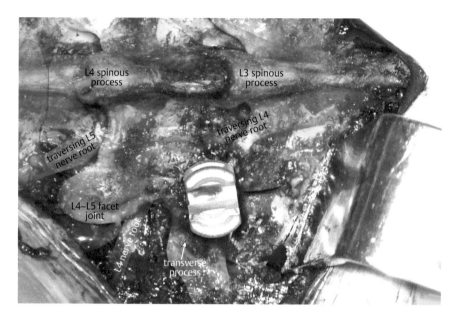

- The pedicle screw is placed.

Potential Pitfalls

Pedicle wall violations and fractures can occur during screw placement, oftentimes with excessive lateral or medial screw placement. Ensure adequate pedicle visualization to avoid screw misplacement.

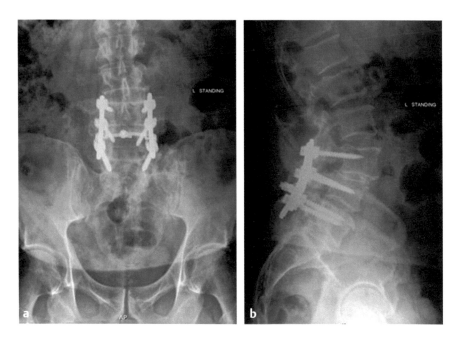

Anteroposterior (a) and lateral (b) postoperative radiographs. Six-month postoperative visit of a patient with L3–L5 posterolateral fusion.

Perioperative Complications

- **Screw misplacement:**
  - Screw positioning beyond the boundaries of the pedicle wall, potentially causing injury to nearby structures including nerve roots, spinal cord:
    - Incidence of approximately 5%.
    - Typically occurs at the pedicle–vertebral body junction (15–20 mm in depth).
  - Characterized by potential back pain, vascular, visceral, neurologic symptoms, or dural tears with possible loss of long-term spinal fixation:
    - Two to eleven percent with screw misplacement experience neurologic dysfunction.
  - Prevention:
    - Increase exposure size through laminectomy or facetectomy if pedicle visualization is difficult.
    - Utilization of preoperative imaging to understand patient's pedicle width and angle and select for appropriate-sized implant.
  - Treatment:
    - If violation occurs, the starting point of the screw can be lateralized and the angulation of the screw can be adjusted.
- **Pedicle fracture:**
  - Fracture of pars interarticularis or pedicle during screw placement, inhibiting proper anchoring of the screw for fixation.
  - Risk factors:
    - Pars interarticularis defect
    - Female sex
    - Smoking
  - Treatment:
    - Some surgeons have suggested using cerclage wire to restore stability, allowing for increased engagement of the screw in the pedicle.

■ Suggested Readings

1. Esses SI, Sachs BL, Dreyzin V. Complications associated with the technique of pedicle screw fixation. A selected survey of ABS members. Spine 1993;18(15):2231–2238, discussion 2238–2239
2. Amato V, Giannachi L, Irace C, Corona C. Accuracy of pedicle screw placement in the lumbosacral spine using conventional technique: computed tomography postoperative assessment in 102 consecutive patients. J Neurosurg Spine 2010;12(3):306–313
3. Lattig F, Fekete TF, Jeszenszky D. Management of fractures of the pedicle after instrumentation with transpedicular screws: A report of three patients. J Bone Joint Surg Br 2010;92(1):98–102

13 Minimally Invasive Lumbar Exposure

- Removal of herniated disks.
- Decompression of nerve roots.
- Posterior lumbar spinal fusions.
- Access to the posterior lumbar spine with minimal blood loss and shortened patient recovery time.

Tips and Pearls before You Begin

Radiographic visualization is extremely important in both the anteroposterior (AP) and lateral views. Often, the initial dilator can be used similar to a Cobb elevator, with gentle subperiosteal dissection being performed to sweep the paraspinal muscle off the lamina. Anatomic landmarks may be difficult to conceptualize as the surgeon adapts to the minimally invasive technique.

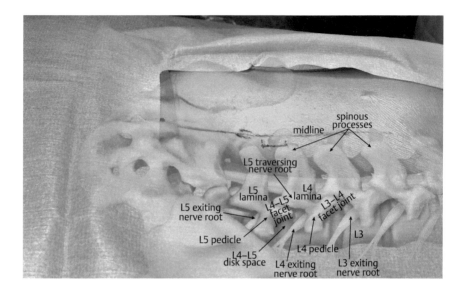

- Through use of an AP fluoroscopic image, key bony landmarks are identified:
  - Midline (spinous processes).
  - Pedicular line (lateral edge of the pedicle).
  - Superior vertebral end plate.
- Skin incision line:
  - For laminectomies, the incision is made closer to the midline.
  - For fusions, the incision is made lateral to the midpedicular line (1.0 cm).
  - The size of the skin incision is dependent on the size of the final working portal (15–26 mm).

Internervous Plane

No true internervous plane is present for minimally invasive lumbar approaches; the entry points are within the paraspinal muscles, which are segmentally innervated.

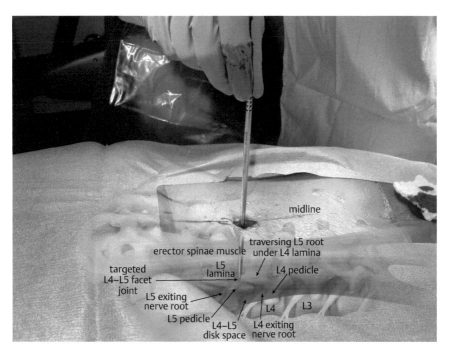

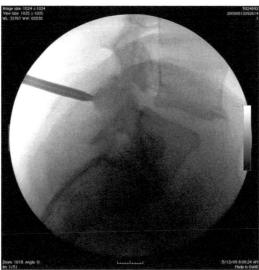

• An initial dilator is used to localize the disk space to be prepared using a lateral fluoroscopic image.

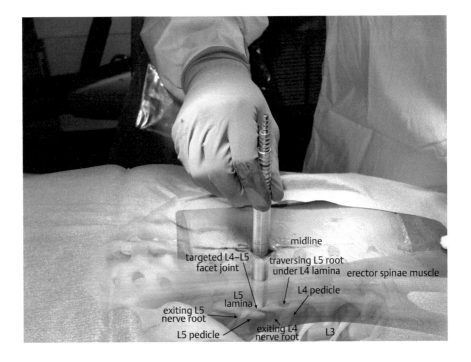

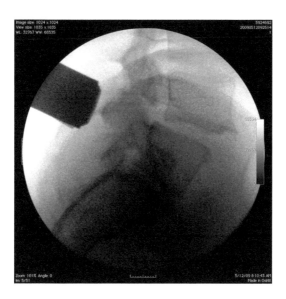

- The dilators are sequentially increased in size, thereby increasing the size of the working portal:
  - The dilators should be gently swept to remove any intervening muscle and soft tissue.

Potential Pitfalls

Incomplete decompression and fusion can occur due to inadequate retractor placement or visualization. Visualization can be improved through the use of radiographic confirmation, meticulous hemostasis, and a rotating surgical table.

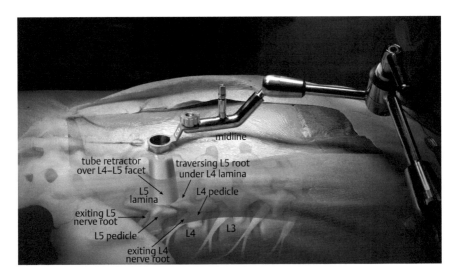

- The final portal is established and firmly connected to the surgical bed.

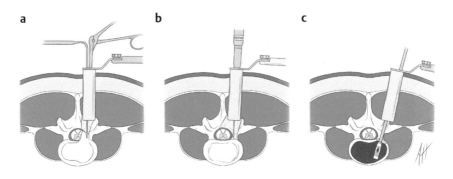

Cross section. Position of the tubular retractors based on intended procedure. **(a)** Minimally invasive diskectomy. **(b)** Minimally invasive laminectomy. **(c)** Minimally invasive transforaminal lumbar interbody fusion.

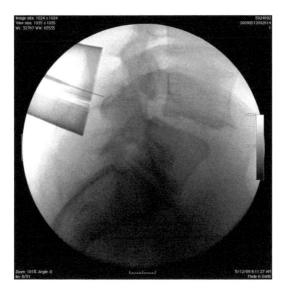

- A lateral fluoroscopic image is obtained to confirm localization of the disk space to be prepared.

14 Minimally Invasive Laminectomy

Proper patient positioning and good **intraoperative imaging** are essential. For the given procedure, it is also important to choose the correct size of the retractor. For a decompression, a smaller diameter retractor is required to allow placement medial to the facet joint. Once the retractor is in the correct position, resist the temptation to move it often because such movement leads to muscle creep into the surgical workspace.

If there is an **incidental durotomy,** it should be treated in a similar fashion to the same complication encountered in an open procedure. A primary suture repair is preferable if it is possible.

Epidural bleeding needs to be proactively controlled. There are several ways to reduce the likelihood of problematic bleeding. First, correct positioning of the patient on the Jackson frame reduces intra-abdominal pressure. When in the epidural space, find the bleeders before they find you and use bipolar electrocautery. Liberally use a thrombotic paste product to minimize bleeding.

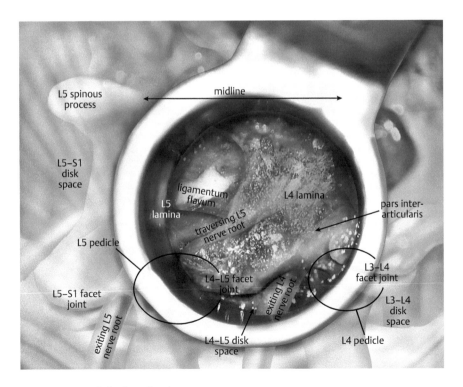

- Exposure of the hemilamina.

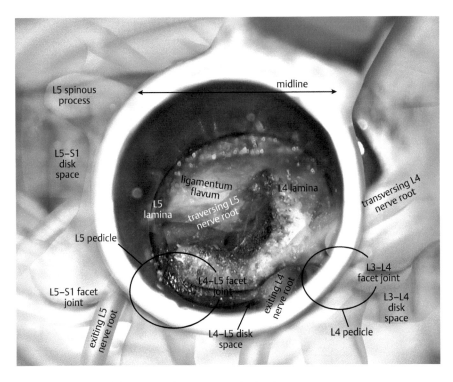

• The high-speed burr is used to remove the lamina.

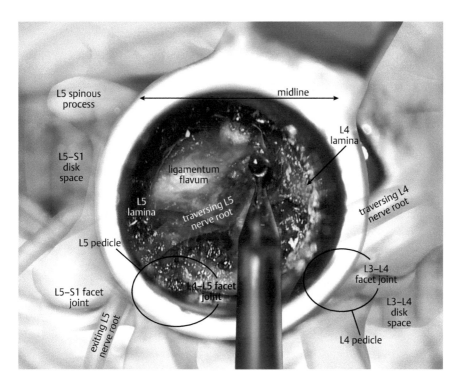

• Undercutting the ipsilateral L4–L5 facet joint.

Potential Pitfalls

Iatrogenic fractures can occur from excessive removal of the **pars interarticu-laris** and the **inferior articular process.** Avoid unnecessary thinning of these structures to prevent fractures or instability.

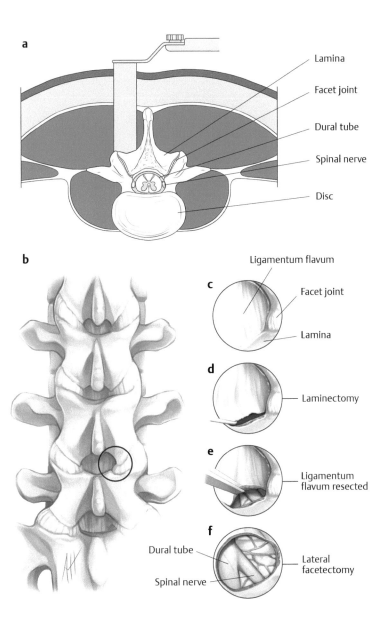

Cross sectional and top-down view of exposure. **(a–b)** The entry point for the exposure is approximately 2 cm from midline, directly overlying the superior lamina and inferior ligamentum flavum of the intended vertebral level. If bilateral decompression needs to be performed, entry point 3 to 4 cm from midline is used to allow for angulation of the retractors to reach the contralateral side. **(c–f)** Removal of the superior lamina, attached ligamentum flavum, and facet joint to expose the underlying dura and nerve root.

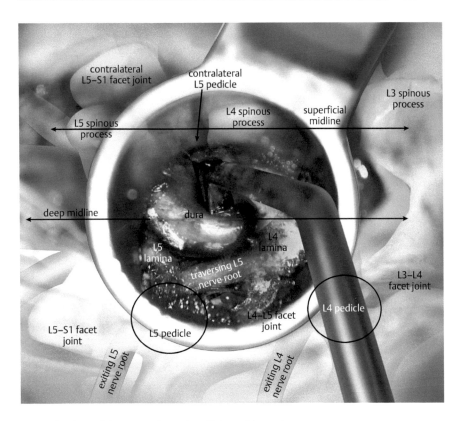

- Palpation of the contralateral pedicle and lateral recess.

Potential Pitfalls

Dural tears can occur with excessive removal of the ligamentum flavum or retraction of dural structures. Repair of dural tears is similar to those that occur during open procedures.

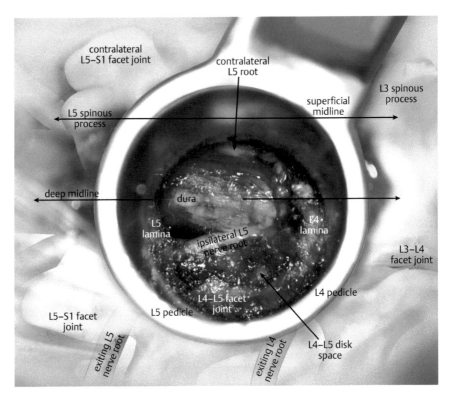

- The decompression occurs with the tube directed medially; therefore, the superficial midline is crossed during the decompression.
- A completed laminectomy demonstrates that the thecal sac is completely compressed, with the overlying paraspinal muscle preserved.

Perioperative Complications[a]

[a]See **Chapter 11: Open Laminectomy and Diskectomy** for common complications that can also occur following minimally invasive lumbar laminectomy.

Suggested Readings

1.   Nerland US, Jakola AS, Solheim O, et al. Minimally invasive decompression versus open laminectomy for central stenosis of the lumbar spine: pragmatic comparative effectiveness study. BMJ 2015;350:h1603

15 Minimally Invasive Far Lateral Diskectomy

Far lateral disk herniations affect the nerve root exiting lateral to the **neurofo-ramen.** Therefore, a standard **hemilaminotomy** will not allow for visualization of the disk herniation without excessive or complete resection of the facet joint. **L5–S1** disk herniations pose an additional anatomic challenge because the sacral ala and iliac wing will often make a far lateral approach more technically demanding.

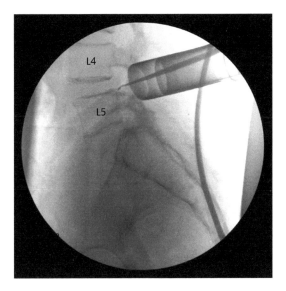

• Lateral fluoroscopic visualization is essential to confirm the appropriate level.

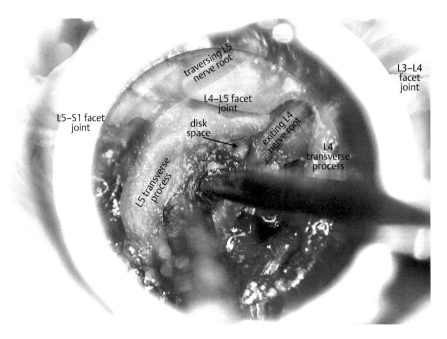

- The incision is typically made 4 cm lateral to the midline. The tube is docked onto the lateral aspect of the pars interarticularis and the inferior transverse process.

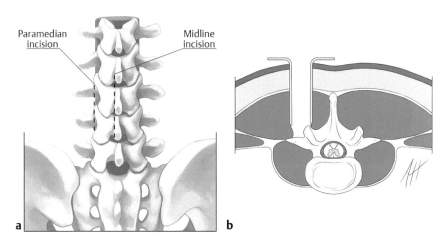

*Anteroposterior **(a)** and cross-sectional view **(b)** of the entry point.* Note the incision placement relative to the typical midline approach. The tubular retractors are placed transmuscularly overlying the facet joint, beyond the neuroforamen.

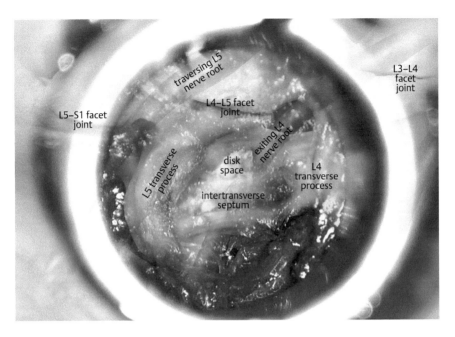

- The tube is docked lateral to the L4–L5 facet joint.

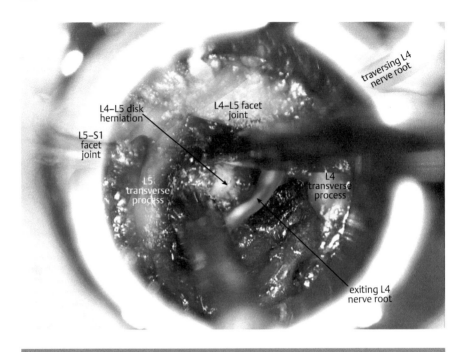

Potential Pitfalls

Significant bleeding can occur during resection of the intertransverse septum. If not controlled, the bleeding can result in inadequate visualization of the herniation and potentially an inadequate decompression.

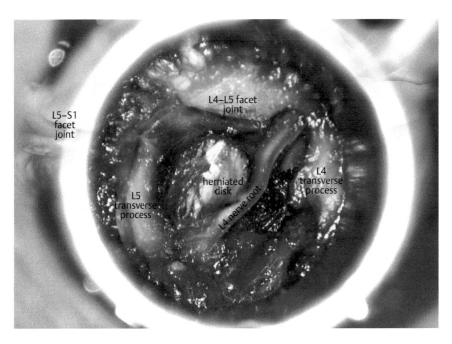

• The nerve root is typically displaced such that it is dorsal and lateral to the disk herniation.

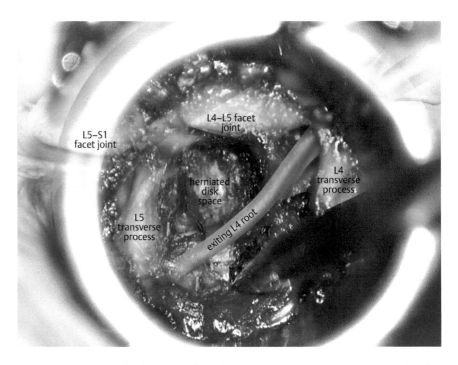

- The nerve root should be gently mobilized superiorly to expose the underlying disk space.

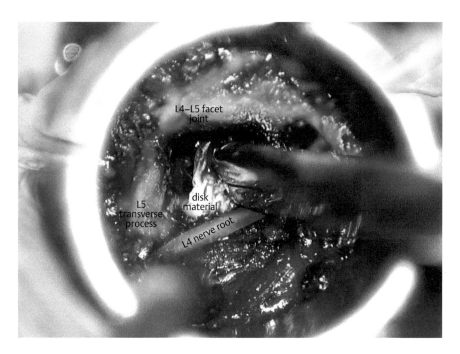

- A pituitary rongeur is used to remove the disk fragments.

Potential Pitfalls

Iatrogenic nerve root injury can occur during mobilization and excision of the herniation. Care should be taken to avoid excessive mobilization of the nerve root.

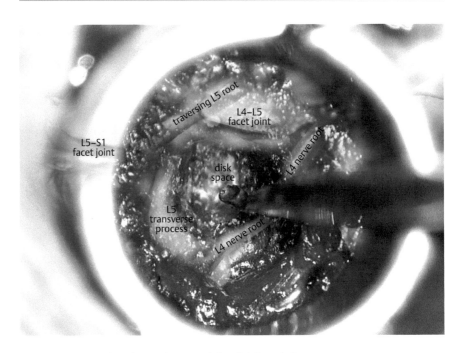

• A curette is placed into the site of the disk herniation.

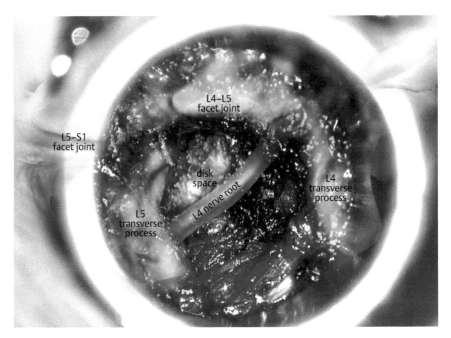

Perioperative Complications[a]

[a]See **Chapter 11: Open Laminectomy and Diskectomy** for common complications also occurring after minimally invasive lumbar far lateral diskectomy.

Suggested Readings

1. Salame K, Lidar Z. Minimally invasive approach to far lateral lumbar disc herniation: technique and clinical results. Acta Neurochir (Wien) 2010;152(4):663–668

16 Minimally Invasive Transforaminal Lumbar Interbody Fusion (TLIF)

Visualization of the disk space is essential. Complete resection of the **facet joint** with removal of all overlying bone from the **superior articular process** of the inferior vertebra should be performed. Disk space preparation is the key to an increased likelihood of a successful arthrodesis. A combination of curettes and Kerrison rongeurs should be used to prepare the end plate. Fluoroscopy may be used to ensure that the **anterior longitudinal ligament** (ALL) is not violated. Care should be taken with paddle distractors and shavers, as these devices may compromise the end plates, which can result in subsidence of the implant.

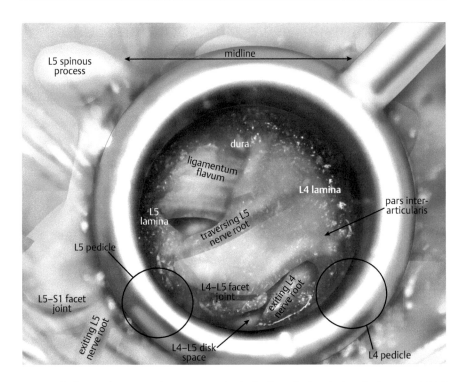

- With the working portal appropriately docked on the level of pathology, an initial exposure can be performed. Often, there are residual paraspinal muscle fibers that must be removed from the lamina.

Potential Pitfalls

Muscle creep can occur under the retractor edges, limiting exposure quality. Care should be taken to remove all soft-tissue structures from the surgical field.

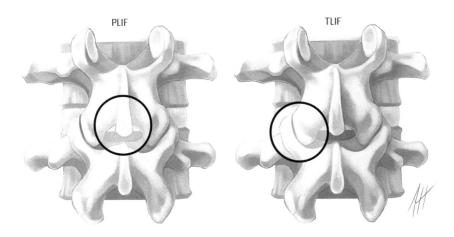

PLIF   TLIF

Anteroposterior view. Working zone for the transforaminal lumbar interbody fusion (TLIF) procedure. Entry point is in between the multifidus and longissimus muscles overlying the lateral facet joint.

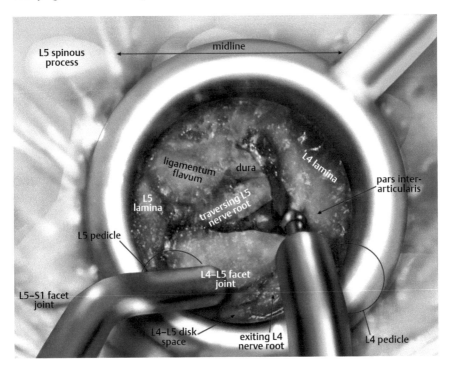

- Once the lamina is exposed, a high-speed burr is used to perform a laminectomy. Bone is removed until only the flavum is visualized:
  - The laminectomy is extended laterally through the pars interarticularis.
  - Bone is saved in a bone trap.

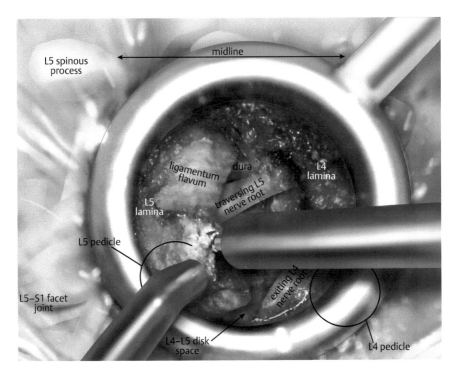

- The laminectomy is extended cranially until the end of the flavum insertion is identified:
  - Epidural fat or dura is often seen.
- This marks the cranial extent of the laminectomy:
  - The burr is then directed directly lateral through the pars interarticularis.

Potential Pitfalls

Pedicle integrity can be compromised during laminectomy and facetectomy. Adequate visualization should be maintained to avoid drilling into the pedicle.

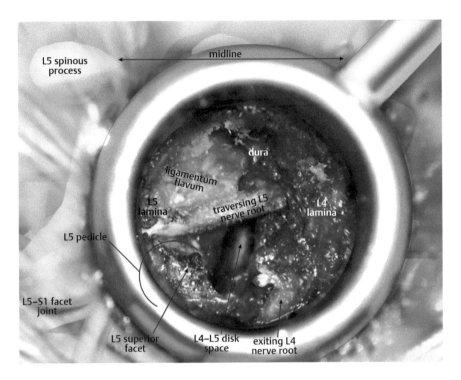

- Once the burr is through the pars, the inferior articular process can be removed, completing the facetectomy and exposing the involved disk space.

Potential Pitfalls

Poor visualization of the disk space and **a narrowed working zone** can result from inadequate resection of the facet joint. Consequently, placement of an undersized implant can occur, increasing the risk of **cage migration and pseudarthrosis.** Ensure complete facet removal before progression to ligamentum flavum resection.

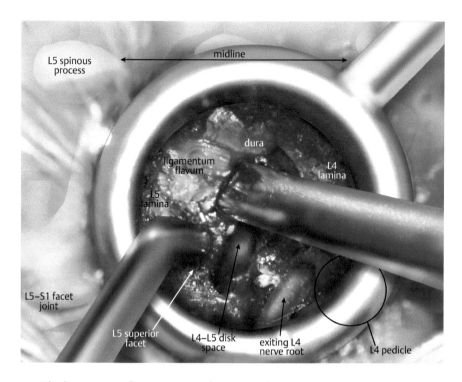

- The ligamentum flavum can now be resected.
- Care is taken to preserve the flavum initially, as it protects the dura while the decompression is being performed.

Potential Pitfalls

Dural tear can occur with overzealous resection of the ligamentum flavum or manipulation of the dura. Avoid removal of the ligamentum flavum until the decompression is completed, especially during contralateral neural decompression.

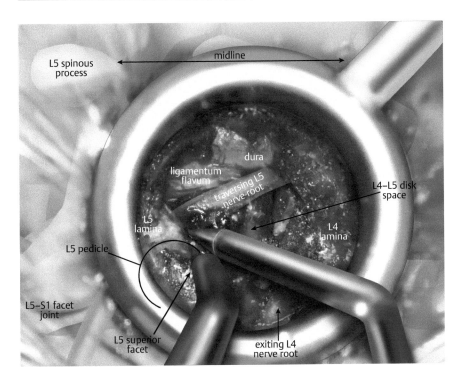

- Bipolar cautery is used to coagulate the veins that overlie the disk space.

Potential Pitfalls

Excessive bleeding and epidural hematoma can result from the bleeding venous plexus surrounding the nerve root and nearby disk. Meticulous cauterization or Gelfoam can be used to mitigate bleeding.

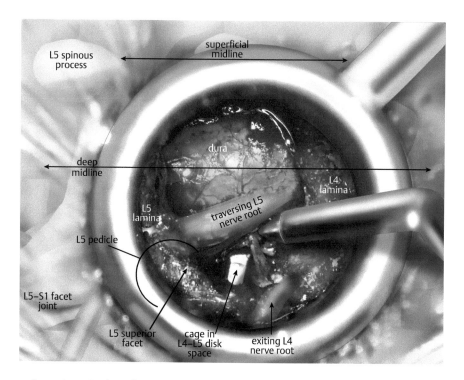

- Once the veins have been coagulated, the inferior pedicle (L5) and disk space (L4–L5) can be visualized:
  – The traversing nerve root (L5) is just medial to the pedicle.
  – The exiting nerve (L4) is above the disk space. It is not typically exposed.

Potential Pitfalls

Nerve root injury can occur from manipulation during disk removal or cage placement. Avoid excessive retraction of nerve root to prevent direct injury.

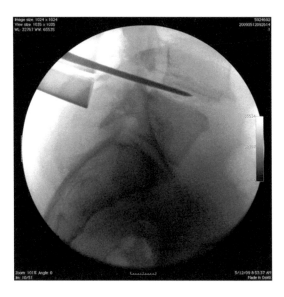

- The working space in the TLIF is lateral to the exiting root in the neuroforamen:
  - Lateral fluoroscopic imaging is used when preparing the disk space.

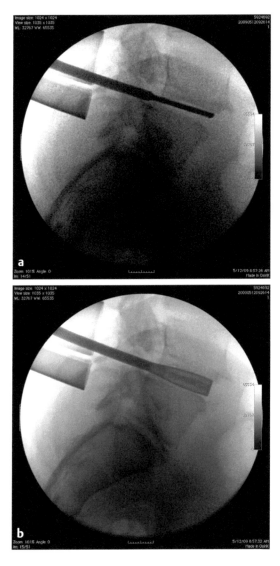

- The disk space is prepared using a combination of paddle distractors and end plate shavers to remove the disk material.

Potential Pitfalls

Incomplete decompression can occur due to a small working area and inadequate visualization. Identification of critical landmarks including the pedicle, pars, and lateral ligamentum flavum is helpful to confirm that all nerve compressions are addressed.

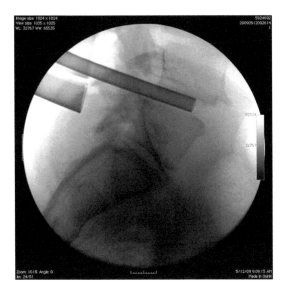

- Once the disk material has been removed and the end plates prepared, a bone funnel is passed into the disk space:
  - The bone collected during the laminectomy can then be placed into the disk space.

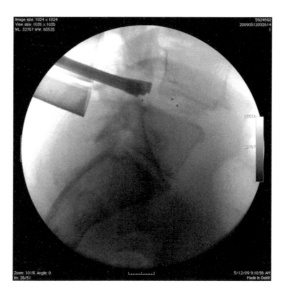

- The interbody cage is then impacted into place:
  - Care is taken to protect the nerve root during cage placement.

Potential Pitfalls

Cage misplacement can result from insufficient disk removal, violation of the bony end plate, or injury to the ALL. Avoid overzealous shaving during disk removal. Fluoroscopic imaging can guide proper end plate preparation and cage placement.

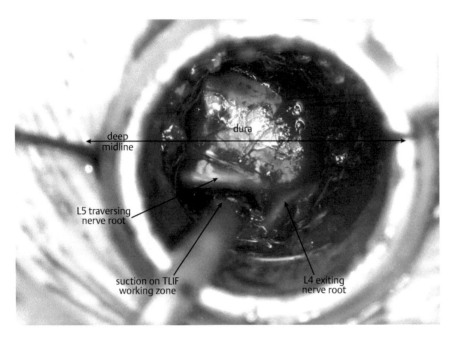

- The interbody cage has been placed into the prepared disk space:
  - The cage is directed obliquely toward the midline.
  The tube can be directed medially to perform a contralateral decompression.

Perioperative Complications

- **Nerve root injury:**
  - Direct damage from manipulation or cage placement, or compression by epidural hematoma:
    - Inferior nerve root more frequently involved.
  - Prevention:
    - Maintain medial-lateral working plane with the tubular retractors.
    - Identification and control of nerve roots in the working zone prior to diskectomy.
- **Dural tears and cerebrospinal fluid (CSF) leak:**
  - Direct damage during decompression or flavum resection:
    - Rare complication due to limited dural exposure in this approach.
  - Prevention:
    - Maintain integrity of flavum during ipsilateral or contralateral neural decompression:
      - Thecal sac protected and pushed ventrally during contralateral work.
  - Treatment:
    - Difficult to repair in this approach.
    - Indirect treatment through collagen sponge or other dural sealant to limit dead space and decrease risk of CSF leakage has been suggested.
- **Cage misplacement and migration:**
  - Insufficient removal of disk, violation of end plate,
  - or injury to ALL resulting in malposition of cage.
  - Characterized by pain and neurologic symptoms depending on location of misplacement.
  - Prevention:
    - Use fluoroscopy to minimize risk of end plate violation or penetration of ALL.
    - Cage placement such that it crosses the midline of the disk space and minimizes the risk of malpositioning.
- **Pseudarthrosis:**
  - Also known as a nonunion.
  - Characterized by persistent pain or neurologic symptoms.
  - Risk factors:
    - Incomplete decompression or disk removal.
    - Inadequate end plate preparation.
    - Inappropriately sized cages.
  - Prevention:
    - Adequate visualization through maximization of working space:
      - Allows for complete decompression and disk removal.
    - Use of insert-and-rotate scrapers to assist in complete disk removal.

▇ Suggested Readings

1. Wong AP, Smith ZA, Nixon AT, et al. Intraoperative and perioperative complications in minimally invasive transforaminal lumbar interbody fusion: a review of 513 patients. J Neurosurg Spine 2015;22(5):487–495
2. Knox JB, Dai JM III, Orchowski J. Osteolysis in transforaminal lumbar interbody fusion with bone morphogenetic protein-2. Spine 2011;36(8):672–676

17 Mini-Open Pedicle Screw Placement

Tips and Pearls before You Begin

Pedicle width increases with caudal progression of the lumbar spine. Two-dimensional fluoroscopy and neuromonitoring should be used to identify pedicle screw trajectory. Maintaining the pedicle screw within the radiologic cortical border of the pedicle will help ensure accurate screw placement.

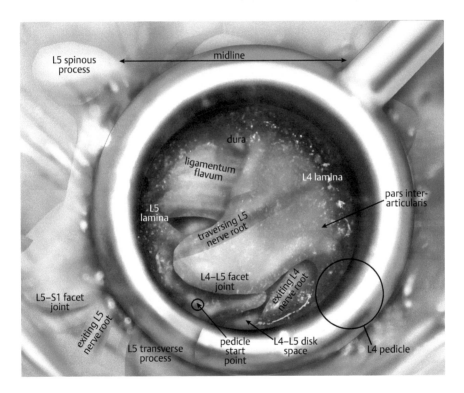

- The pedicle start point is identified through the working portal. This allows for medial–lateral orientation in the anteroposterior (AP) plane.

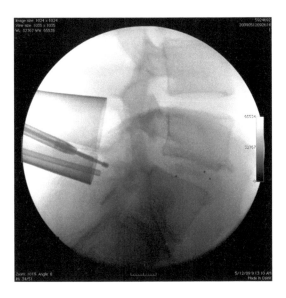

- Lateral fluoroscopic imaging is used to confirm the direction in the cephalad–caudal plane.

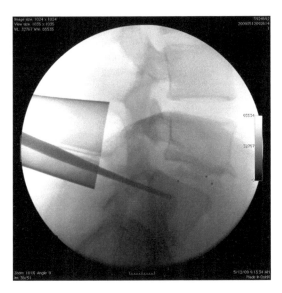

- A gear shift is placed through the pedicle start point to the desired depth under direct lateral fluoroscopy.

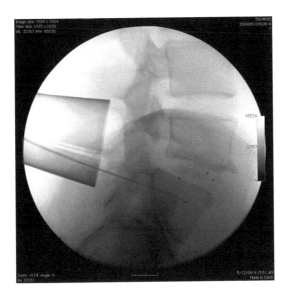

- The pedicle tract is probed.

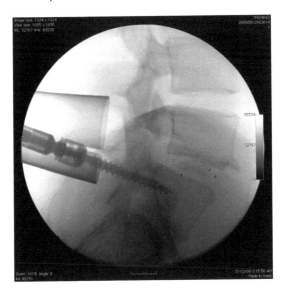

- Pedicle screws are then placed.

Potential Pitfalls

Pedicle violation or breach can occur during screw placement. Meticulous usage of biplanar fluoroscopy is crucial in preventing medial and lateral pedicle breach.

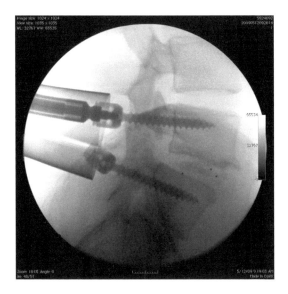

- The same steps are repeated for the adjacent level.

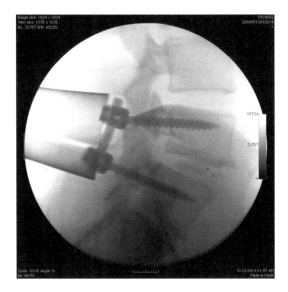

- A rod is then placed and secured through the tube.

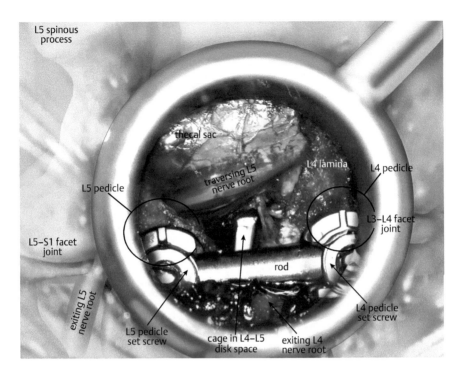

- Intraoperative view.

Perioperative Complications

- **Pedicle violation:**
  - Caused by malpositioning of screws in the anterior, medial, lateral, or inferior direction.
  - Incidence of 0.71 to 4.68%.
  - Presents with:
    - Nerve root or spinal cord injury (medial or inferior violation).
    - Injuries to the aorta, segmental vessels, lung parenchyma, pneumothorax (lateral violation).
    - Injuries to the aorta, vena cava, esophagus (anterior violation).
  - Prevention:
    - Screw placement confirmation with intraoperative AP and lateral radiographs, fluoroscopy, or computed tomography (CT) scan.
    - Postoperative CT scan can confirm placement of the screws and integrity of nearby visceral and neurovascular structures.
- **Screw pullout/failure of fixation:**
  - Caused by malpositioned pedicle screws.
  - Prevention:
    - Use of screw augmentation via polymethylmethacrylate, hydroxyapatite, calcium phosphate, or carbonated apatite in at-risk patients.

■ Suggested Readings

1. Soriano-Sánchez JA, Ortega-Porcayo LA, Gutiérrez-Partida CF, et al. Fluoroscopy-guided pedicle screw accuracy with a mini-open approach: a tomographic evaluation of 470 screws in 125 patients. Int J Spine Surg 2015;9:54
2. Robertson PA, Stewart NR. The radiologic anatomy of the lumbar and lumbosacral pedicles. Spine 2000;25(6):709–715

18 Percutaneous Pedicle Screw Placement

Tips and Pearls before You Begin

As direct visualization of the vital anatomic structures are not possible, it is imperative that unobstructed imaging be obtained to best guide instrumentation placement. Thus, adequate patient positioning must be evaluated prior to draping. The spinal regions of interest should not overlie areas of the operating table where C-arm access is difficult.

Superficial landmarks include:

- Gluteal cleft
- Thoracic and lumbar spinous processes:
  - Appropriate level **must** be confirmed via fluoroscopic imaging.

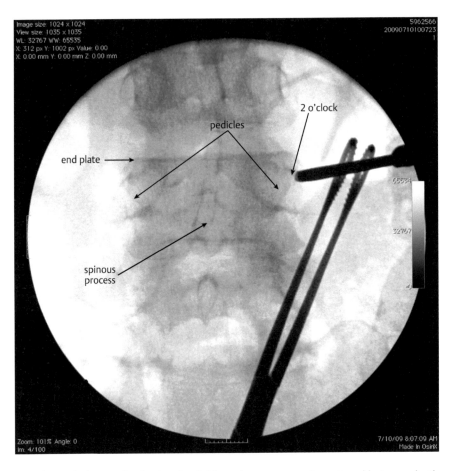

- The end plate is clearly visualized. The spinous process is centered between both pedicles. The Jamshidi needle is started at the 2 o'clock position.

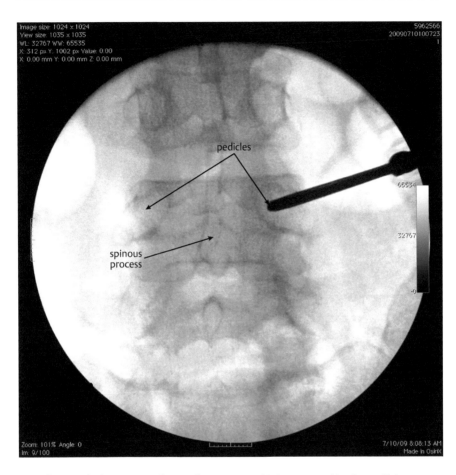

- The Jamshidi trocar is advanced 15 mm until it is centered in the pedicle.

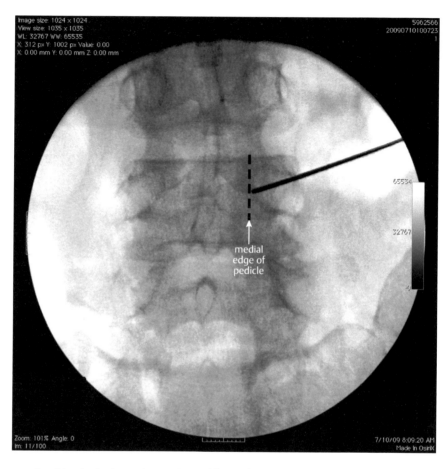

medial
edge of
pedicle

- A guidewire is then advanced an additional 10 mm until it abuts the medial wall of the pedicle on the anteroposterior (AP) image.

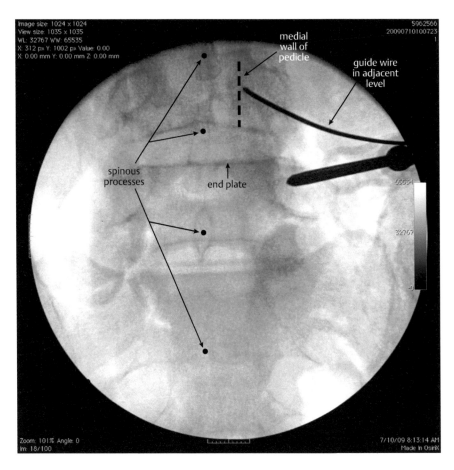

- The steps are repeated for the adjacent level. End plate visualization and centering the spinous process are essential steps for ensuring accurate percutaneous screw placement.

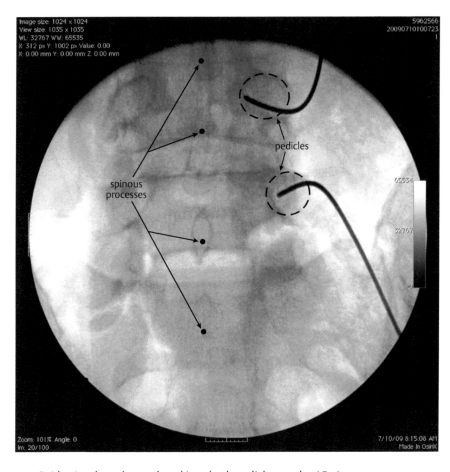

• Guidewires have been placed into both pedicles on the AP view.

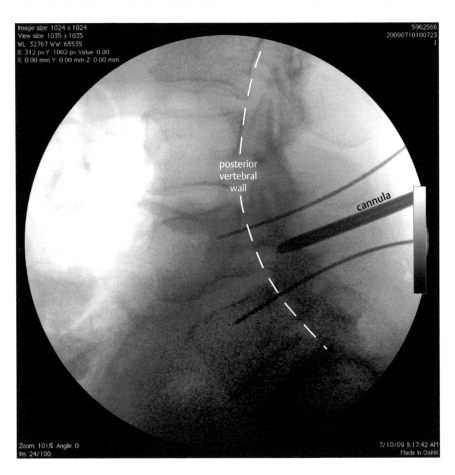

- A lateral image is then obtained to confirm that the guidewires are past the vertebral body wall. This image is extremely important, as it confirms that the guidewire has not breached the medial wall of the pedicle before entrance into the vertebral body. A cannula is then placed in between the guidewires.

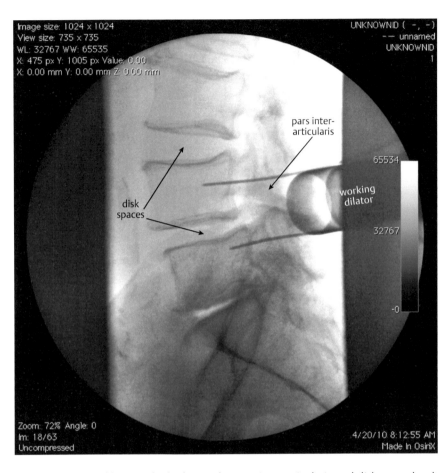

- The working dilator is docked over the pars interarticularis and disk space level. The disk space is prepared as previously described.

Potential Pitfalls

Guidewire pullout is a concern during all remaining steps of the procedure. Ensure adequate advancement of the guidewire past the posterior border of the vertebral body with fluoroscopic imaging.

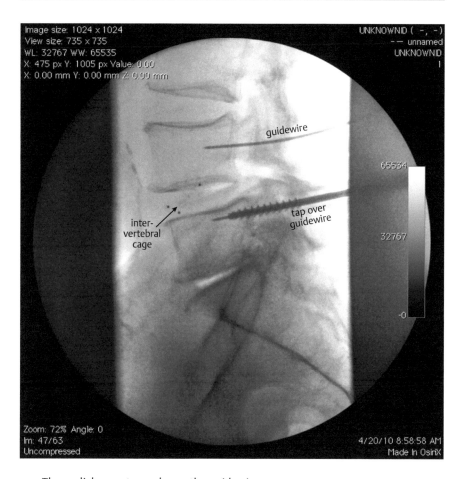

* The pedicles are tapped over the guidewire.

Potential Pitfalls

Loss of guidewire control can lead to entry of the wire into the peritoneum. Taking regular lateral fluoroscopic images helps to avoid inadvertent advancement during tapping or screw placement.

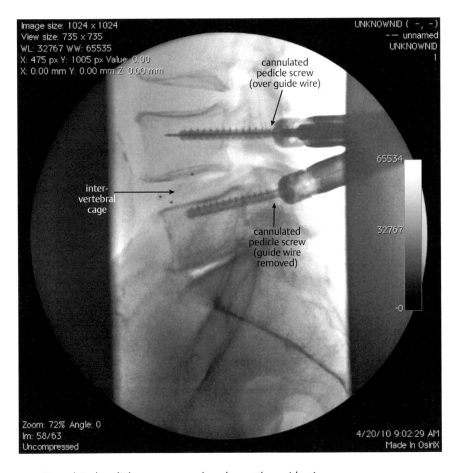

• Cannulated pedicle screws are placed over the guidewire.

Potential Pitfalls

Difficulty with initial pedicle cannulation can lead to **pedicle violation.** Take numerous images with high-quality fluoroscopy to ensure no violation has occurred.

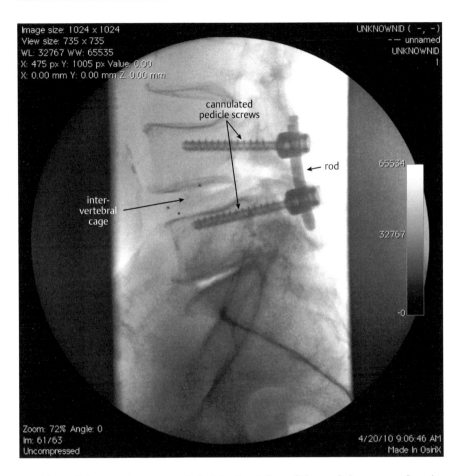

• The rod is passed submuscularly into the tulips of the pedicle screws after the guidewires are removed. Gentle compression can be applied to the graft.

Potential Pitfalls

Pedicle violation can occur with misplacement of the pedicle screws. Prior to locking the construct, imaging should be obtained to ensure all screw heads are in the correct anatomic position.

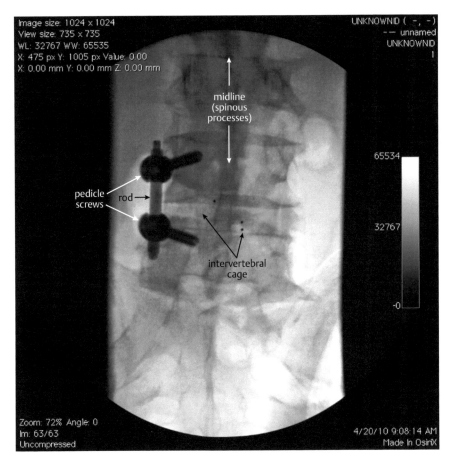

• Final AP image, demonstrating centered cage placement and gently converging pedicle screws.

Perioperative Complications

- **Loss of guidewire control or guidewire pullout:**
  - Caused by initial malpositioning or changes in position during tapping or pedicle screw placement.
  - Prevention:
    - Ensure adequate advancement of the wire past the posterior border of the vertebral body.
    - Mark the guidewire before tapping or screw placement to help indicate unintended advancement.
- **Pedicle violation:**
  - Caused by malpositioning of screws in the anterior, medial, lateral, or inferior direction.
  - Presents with:
    - Nerve root or spinal cord injury (medial or inferior violation).
    - Injuries to the aorta, segmental vessels, lung parenchyma, pneumothorax (lateral violation).
    - Injuries to the aorta, vena cava, esophagus (anterior violation).
  - Prevention:
    - Screw placement confirmation with intraoperative AP and lateral radiographs, fluoroscopy, or computed tomography (CT) scan.
    - Postoperative CT scan can confirm placement of the screws and integrity of nearby visceral and neurovascular structures.
- **Screw pullout/failure of fixation:**
  - Caused by malpositioned pedicle screws.
  - Prevention:
    - Use of screw augmentation via polymethylmethacrylate, hydroxyapatite, calcium phosphate, or carbonated apatite in at-risk patients.

■ Suggested Readings

1. Bydon M, Xu R, Amin AG, et al. Safety and efficacy of pedicle screw placement using intraoperative computed tomography: consecutive series of 1148 pedicle screws. J Neurosurg Spine 2014;21(3):320–328
2. Gautschi OP, Schatlo B, Schaller K, Tessitore E. Clinically relevant complications related to pedicle screw placement in thoracolumbar surgery and their management: a literature review of 35,630 pedicle screws. Neurosurg Focus 2011;31(4):E8

19 Extreme (eXtreme) Lateral Interbody Fusion

▇ Lateral Lumbar

- Spinal fusion
- Corpectomy
- Diskectomy
- Vertebral body biopsy
- Psoas abscess drainage
- Curettage of infected vertebral bodies

▇ Positioning

Positioning of lateral lumbar procedures is similar to that of lateral thoracic procedures. Please refer to **Chapter 9: Minimally Invasive Thoracic Corpectomy** for detailed positioning instructions.

Superficial landmarks include:

- Twelfth rib
- Pubic symphysis
- Lateral border of the rectus abdominis:
  – Five centimeters lateral to the midline

Tips and Pearls before You Begin

A good fluoroscopic image is extremely helpful. Adjust the surgical table such that cephalocaudal angle of the C-arm is perpendicular to the floor. There is a tendency to cheat the initial exposure anterior to avoid the nerves posteriorly. However, because the retractor is designed to prevent pressure on the posterior elements, the aperture is preferentially expanded anteriorly. Therefore, the ideal initial target spot is the **direct center of the lateral aspect of the disk**, which will result in retractor exposure of the anterior half of the disk space. Multilevel procedures can be performed with the same skin incision but separate fascial incisions and psoas muscle dilations. In **degenerative scoliosis cases**, coronal alignment can be achieved from either side, but access is typically easier from the concave side, which allows access to multiple levels through the same incision. The contralateral annulus must be disrupted to achieve parallel distraction, optimal biomechanical position of the implant, and optimal coronal alignment.

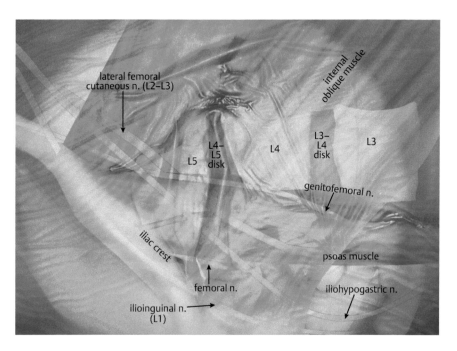

- The patient is placed into a direct lateral position.
- It is essential that the patient be directly perpendicular to the ground to ensure true anteroposterior (AP) and lateral fluoroscopic views of the disk space.
- AP and lateral fluoroscopic imaging is used to identify the disk space.

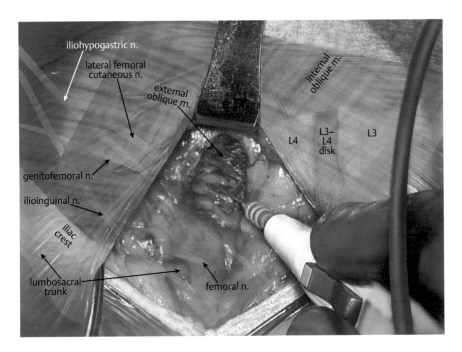

• A skin incision is made, exposing the fibers of the external oblique muscle.

Internervous Plane

There is no internervous plane in this approach. The muscles of the abdominal wall, which are divided in line with the skin incision, are segmentally innervated. No significant denervation occurs.

Potential Pitfalls

Avoid prolonged retraction time to avoid neuropraxia to the lumbar plexus. Suggested operative time per level should be less than 20 minutes to minimize the risk of lumbar plexus neuropraxia.

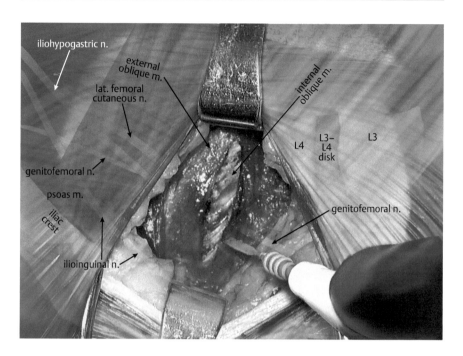

- The fibers of the internal oblique muscle lie underneath the external oblique:
  - These fibers run in opposite directions.

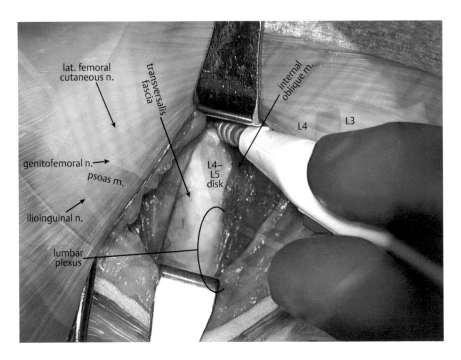

- Once the fibers of the internal oblique are split, the transversalis fascia is identified.

Potential Pitfalls

Visceral injury (perforation, great vessel injury, kidney-ureteral injury) can occur during exposure before placement of the retractors. Meticulous finger dissection should occur prior to retractor insertion to identify and protect viscera by sweeping the retroperitoneum and its contents anteriorly.

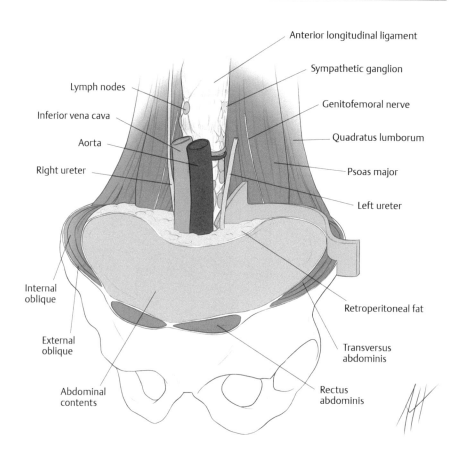

Anterior longitudinal ligament

Sympathetic ganglion

Lymph nodes

Genitofemoral nerve

Inferior vena cava

Aorta

Quadratus lumborum

Right ureter

Psoas major

Left ureter

Internal oblique

Retroperitoneal fat

External oblique

Transversus abdominis

Abdominal contents

Rectus abdominis

Anatomic exposure illustrating relationship of visceral structures to the anterior vertebral bodies. The interval between the psoas and aorta allows access to the anterior vertebral bodies for fusion (*green arrow*).

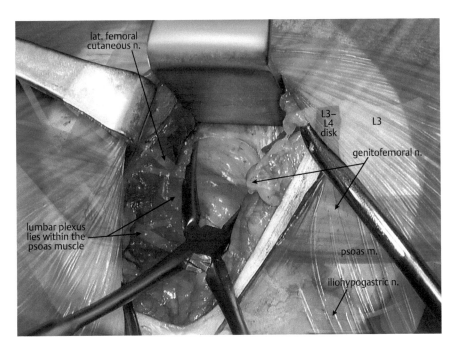

- The transversalis fascia is bluntly opened, exposing the retroperitoneal fat.

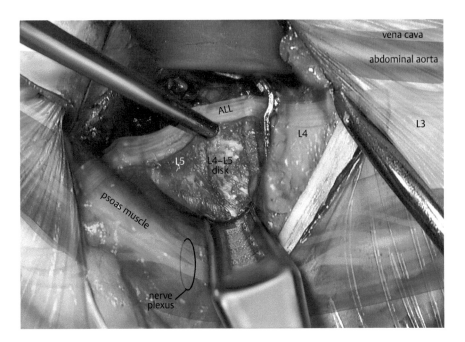

- The psoas muscle is then identified. It can be either traversed with continuous neuromonitoring or swept posteriorly.
- The lumbar plexus lies within the substance of the psoas, so care should be taken to avoid the lumbar nerve roots, particularly at the L4–L5 level.
- Bipolar cautery is used to expose the disk space, removing any residual overlying fibers of the psoas muscle.

Potential Pitfalls

Neural injury, especially to the **lumbosacral plexus or sympathetic ganglion**, can occur with manipulation of the psoas. Use of neuromonitoring can aid in mapping nerve locations. Redirection of the approach may be necessary if ventral nerves are encountered.

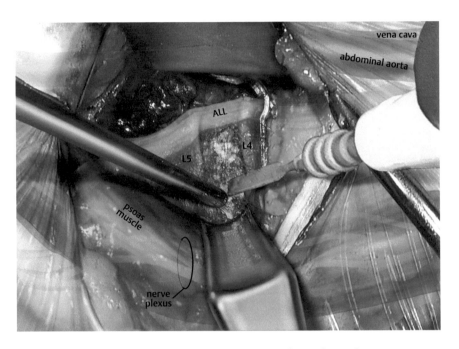

- Once the disk space is exposed, an annulotomy can be performed:
  - Note that the nerve root is posterior to the posterior retractor blade.

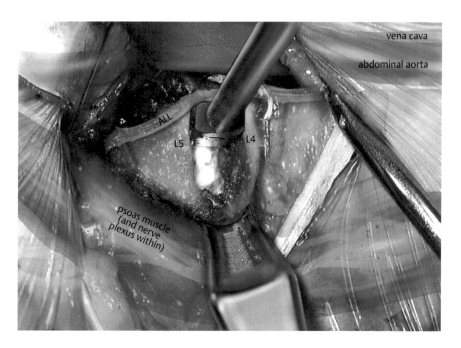

- The end plate is carefully prepared, with particular attention to avoiding violation of the vertebral end plates.
- It is essential to prepare the entire end plate across the contralateral side:
  - Releasing the contralateral annulus will greatly improve exposure and allow for correction of coronal plane deformities.

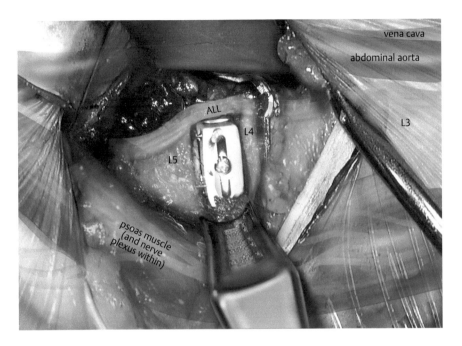

- An intervertebral cage is gently impacted into place:
  - The cage should span the entire width of the vertebral body, thereby resting on the ring apophysis.
    - This placement will minimize the likelihood of cage subsidence.
- The cage is placed using AP and lateral fluoroscopic imaging.

Potential Pitfalls

Subsidence or cage malpositioning can occur with improper cage size or placement. Ensure that end plates are prepared adequately and that no violations occur.

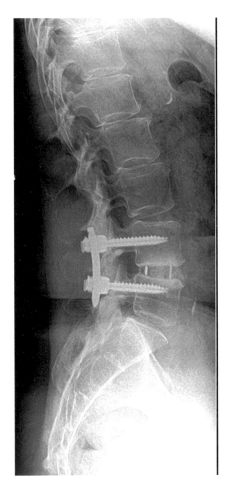

Lateral view. Postoperative radiograph showing placement of an interbody cage after lateral lumbar interbody fusion at L4–L5. Note the presence of unilateral pedicle screws in L4–L5, as well.

Perioperative Complications

- **Visceral injury:**
  - Caused by manipulation of tissues during initial exposure and retractor placement.
  - Presents with abdominal viscera perforation, injury to the great vessels, kidney-ureteral injury, psoas/retroperitoneal hematoma, or rhabdomyolysis.
  - Prevention:
    - Before insertion of dilators/retractors, meticulous finger dissection is required to palpate visceral structures and to sweep the retroperitoneum and its contents anteriorly.
    - Any structures present within the surgical field should be swept posteriorly or held posterior to the dilator/retractor.
- **Neural injury:**
  - Occurs with traversal of the psoas muscle or direct injury to the lumbosacral plexus or sympathetic ganglion.
  - Presents with hip flexor weakness, thigh numbness, genitofemoral neuralgia:
    - Temporary neurologic deficit—9.40% of cases.
    - Permanent neurologic deficit—2.46% of cases.
  - Prevention:
    - Neuromonitoring is used to map nerve locations and redirect the approach as necessary if nerves are encountered.
    - In multilevel cases, allow muscle and nerves to relax intermittently.
- **Subsidence/coronal imbalance:**
  - Caused by improper technique in end plate preparation or with use of an inappropriately sized implant.
  - Prevention:
    - Proper technique in end plate preparation, avoidance of end plate violations.
    - Wider implants with greater surface area are resistant to subsidence.

◼ Suggested Readings

1. Grimm BD, Leas DP, Poletti SC, Johnson DR II. Postoperative complications within the first year after extreme lateral interbody fusion: experience of the first 108 patients. Clin Spine Surg 2016;29(3):E151–E156
2. Härtl R, Joeris A, McGuire RA. Comparison of the safety outcomes between two surgical approaches for anterior lumbar fusion surgery: anterior lumbar interbody fusion (ALIF) and extreme lateral interbody fusion (ELIF). Eur Spine J 2016;25(5):1484–1521

20 Minimally Invasive Lumbar Corpectomy

Tips and Pearls before You Begin

The approach for the minimally invasive lumbar corpectomy is similar to that of the extreme lateral interbody fusion. However, care should be taken to be more anterior to the **psoas muscle,** because two disk space levels are treated simultaneously, which increases the likelihood of postoperative lumbar nerve root dysfunction. The upper lumbar levels (L1–L3) are much easier to treat because the psoas is less prominent at these levels and the retractor can be safely positioned anterior to the psoas. At the L4 vertebral level, the patient should be informed that there may be a chance for **postoperative psoas** and **lower lumbar nerve root dysfunction.** In the majority of cases, the dysfunction resolves within 2 to 4 weeks postoperatively.

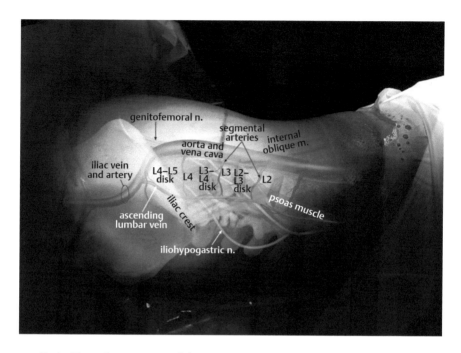

- Typical lateral positioning of the patient.

Superficial landmarks include:

- Twelfth rib.
- Pubic symphysis.
- Lateral border of the rectus abdominis:
  - Five centimeters lateral to the midline.

Internervous Plane

There is no internervous plane in this approach. The muscles of the abdominal wall, which are divided in line with the skin incision, are segmentally innervated. No significant denervation occurs.

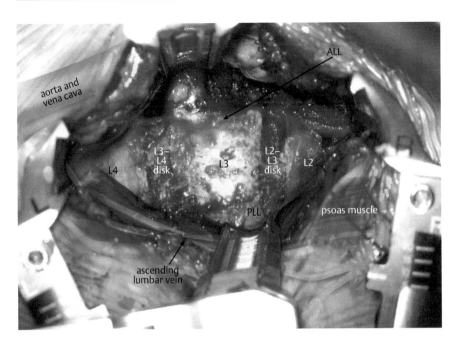

- The dilator has been docked over the pathologic vertebral body. The psoas is retracted posteriorly.

Potential Pitfalls

Nerve injury to the lumbosacral plexus or sympathetic ganglion can occur during initial exposure and dissection toward the vertebral body. Neuromonitoring and diligent fluoroscopy is necessary to determine proximity to nerves and any subsequent alterations to the approach.

Potential Pitfalls

Injury to the **segmental artery** can occur upon exposure of the vertebral body. Expeditious identification and ligation of this artery can prevent unnecessary hemorrhage.

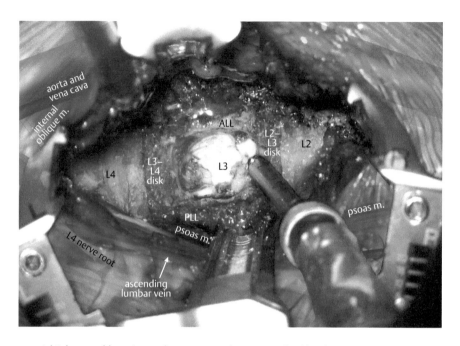

• A high-speed burr is used to remove the L3 vertebral body.

Potential Pitfalls

Visceral injury, such as that to the great vessels, can occur with improper retractor placement during many parts of the procedure. The anterior border of the retractor must be placed appropriately to protect the great vessels and abdominal viscera.

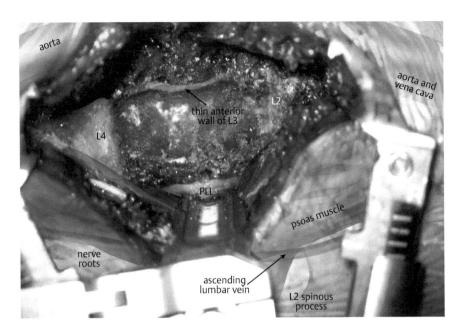

• The corpectomy is complete. The L2–L3 and L3–L4 disk spaces have been resected. The L3 vertebral body has been removed, leaving only a thin wall and the posterior longitudinal ligament intact.

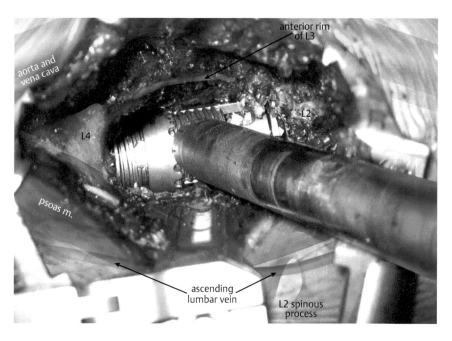

- An expandable titanium cage is appropriately sized and distracted until a press fit is obtained.

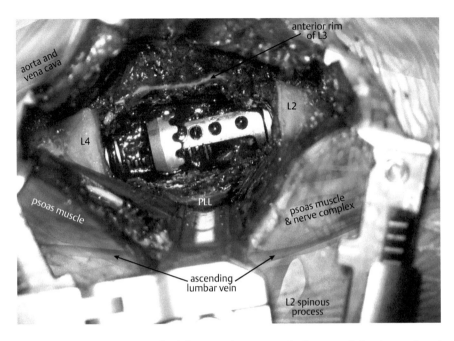

- The cage is shown in its final distracted position. The bone graft has been placed inside and around the cage.

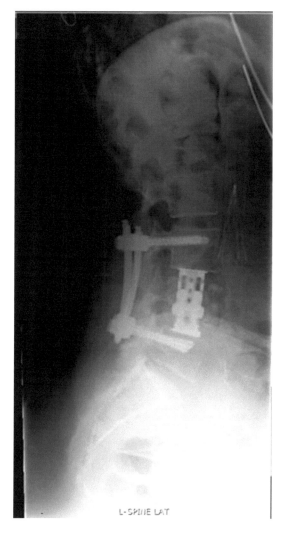

Lateral view. Postoperative radiograph showing placement of an interbody cage after corpectomy at L4. Note the presence of bilateral pedicle screws and rods indicative of an associated fixation as well.

Perioperative Complications

- **Visceral injury:**
  - Caused by manipulation of tissues during initial exposure and retractor placement.
  - Presents with abdominal viscera perforation, injury to the great vessels, kidney-ureteral injury, psoas/retroperitoneal hematoma, or rhabdomyolysis.
  - Prevention:
    - Adequate placement of the anterior portion of the retractor to ensure protection of visceral structures.
- **Segmental artery injury:**
  - Occurs during exposure of the vertebral body, usually during the third pass through the psoas muscle.
  - Presents with hemorrhage.
  - Treatment:
    - Hemostasis via ligation or thrombotic agents (i.e., Gelfoam).
- **Neural injury:**
  - Occurs with traversal of the psoas muscle leading to direct injury to the lumbosacral plexus or sympathetic ganglion. Transient symptoms may also be due to muscle retraction with dilators.
  - Presents with hip flexor weakness, thigh numbness, genitofemoral neuralgia.
  - Treatment:
    - Often self-resolves within 6 months.
  - Prevention:
    - Neuromonitoring and diligent fluoroscopy is used to map nerve locations and redirect the approach as necessary if nerves are encountered.

■ Suggested Readings

1. Adkins DE, Sandhu FA, Voyadzis JM. Minimally invasive lateral approach to the thoracolumbar junction for corpectomy. J Clin Neurosci 2013;20(9):1289–1294
2. Baaj AA, Dakwar E, Le TV, et al. Complications of the mini-open anterolateral approach to the thoracolumbar spine. J Clin Neurosci 2012;19(9):1265–1267

21 Anterior Lumbar Interbody Fusion

■ Anterior Lumbar Positioning

- Lumbar fusion at lower lumbar levels:
  - L4–L5
  - L5–S1

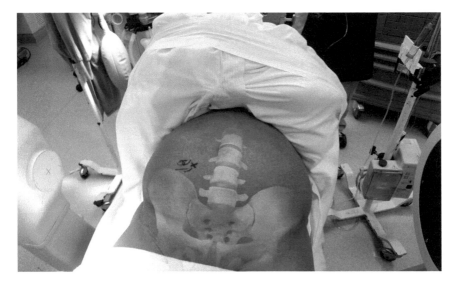

The patient is positioned with his or her arms across the chest. This allows for the C-arm to be moved cephalad in the field. A lateral C-arm is essential for localization and implant placement.

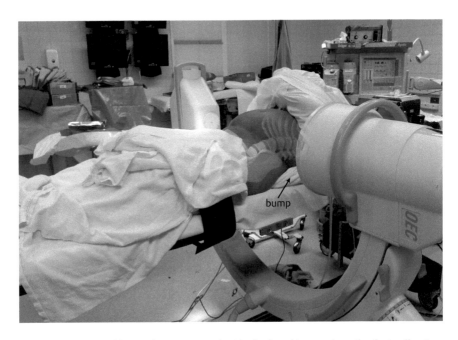

Additionally, the table can be positioned with the head lower than the feet, allowing the abdominal contents to fall away from the operative field. A bump may be placed under the sacrum to increase lordosis.

Superficial landmarks include:

- Umbilicus:
  - Opposite the L3–L4 disk space.
- Pubic symphysis:
  - Pubic tubercle—upper border of pubic symphysis located lateral to the midline.

Tips and Pearls before You Begin

Lateral fluoroscopy is helpful during preoperative localization. Localization will help to minimize tissue dissection and reduce surgical time. Lateral fluoroscopy is also beneficial during implant placement. The **ideal implant position** is a few millimeters recessed deep to the anterior margin of the adjacent end plates. The osteophytes should be rongeured off the anterior end plates before the diskectomy, as they may obscure normal anatomy and result in improper placement of the interbody implant. Once the **anterior annulus** is incised, a Cobb elevator may be used to detach the Sharpey fibers from the superior and inferior end plates, and then the disk can be removed in one piece. **Overly sclerotic end plates** can be burred to expose the bleeding end plates. Sequential dilation of the disk space with sizers is an important step to distract the end plates adequately and insert a press-fit implant.

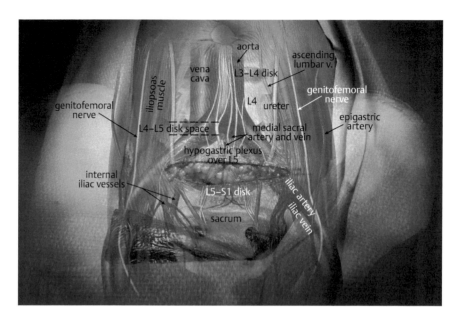

A lateral fluoroscopic image should be obtained before incision to localize the surgical level. At the L4–L5 disk space level, the great vessels are retracted to the right. At L4–L5, the ascending lumbar vein may need to be ligated to mobilize the vessels. Once the incision has been made, the fascia of the rectus abdominis muscle is incised. The fascial incision can be made either horizontally (in line with the skin incision) or vertically, depending on the surgeon's preference.

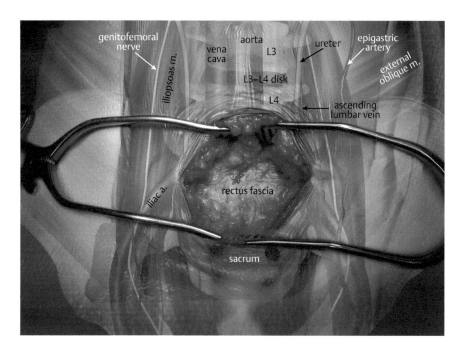

• Rectus fascia incised.

Internervous Plane

The 7th to 12th intercostal nerves segmentally innervate the abdominal musculature. As a result, a midline incision is within the internervous plane.

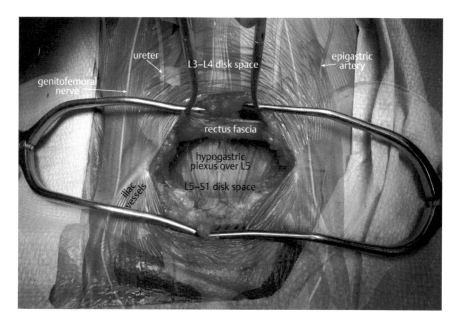

- The muscle belly of the rectus is mobilized. Some surgeons argue that mobilizing the lateral edge of the rectus results in denervation of the muscle, while others state that medial mobilization increases the likelihood for abdominal hernias. Posterior to the rectus is the rectus sheath, which is incised carefully, exposing the retroperitoneum.

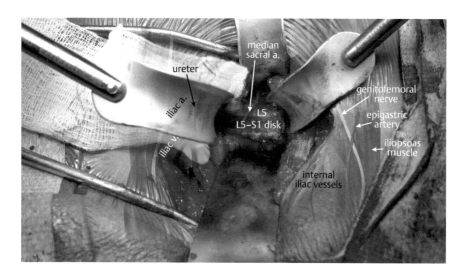

Potential Pitfalls

Nerve injury to the presacral plexus can lead to retrograde ejaculation and impotence. Avoid use of monopolar cautery in the presacral region.

Potential Pitfalls

Middle sacral artery injury can lead to hemorrhage. Prevention entails identification and ligation of the vessel.

Potential Pitfalls

Visceral injury to the ureters or great vessels can occur during dissection. Careful attention must be taken to identify and laterally retract these structures.

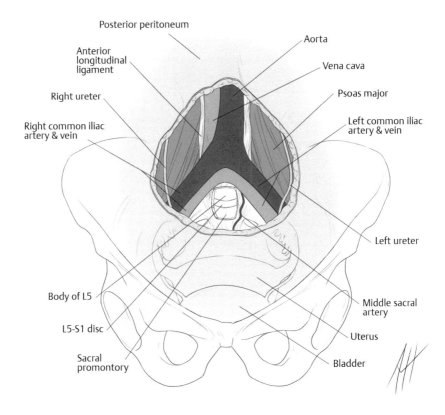

Posterior peritoneum

Anterior
longitudinal
ligament

Right ureter

Right common iliac
artery & vein

Aorta

Vena cava

Psoas major

Left common iliac
artery & vein

Left ureter

Body of L5

L5-S1 disc

Sacral
promontory

Middle sacral
artery

Uterus

Bladder

Coronal view. The exposed L5–S1 disk space is shown, along with its relationship to visceral structures such as the great vessels, psoas major, ureters, and sacral promontory.

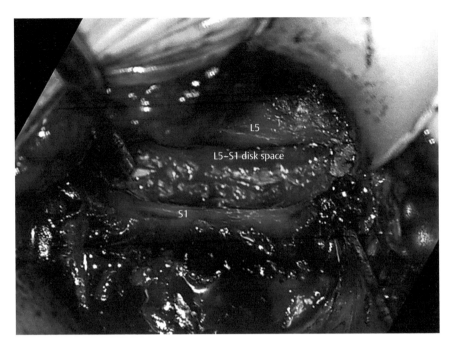

- Once the disk space is identified, an annulotomy can be made with either a knife or an electrocautery device. This procedure is similar to the end plate preparation performed during an anterior cervical diskectomy and fusion.

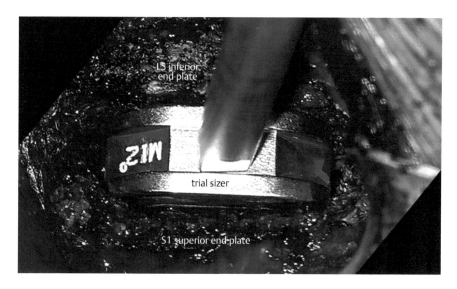

• Care is taken to preserve the integrity of the vertebral end plate. End plate violation may result in implant subsidence and migration. Lateral fluoroscopy should be used to recess the implant below the level of the anterior vertebral margin.

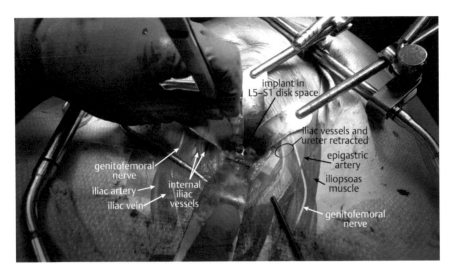

- Often, it is helpful to identify the midline prior to making the annulotomy, thereby ensuring the appropriate positioning of the implant in the anteroposterior direction.

Potential Pitfalls

Subsidence, end plate fracture, or graft displacement can occur, resulting from poor exposure or inadequate disk space preparation leading to improper cage placement or size selection.

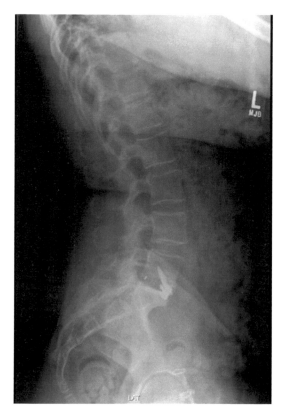

Lateral view. Postoperative radiograph showing placement of an interbody cage after anterior lumbar interbody fusion at L5–S1.

Perioperative Complications

- **Presacral plexus nerve injury:**
  - Caused by manipulation of the presacral plexus adjacent to the L5–S1 levels.
  - Presents with:
    - Retrograde ejaculation with or without impotence.
  - Prevention:
    - Ensure midline incision is long enough for adequate nerve mobilization.
    - Avoid use of monopolar electrocautery in this region.
- **Great vessel injury:**
  - Caused by improper handling and retraction of the great vessels during exposure.
  - Presents with significant hemorrhage, possible death.
  - Treatment:
    - Hemostasis and primary suture or double ligature repair.
    - Vascular surgery consultation.
  - Prevention:
    - Ligation of penetrating lumbar vessels allows for more effective retraction of the great vessels.
- **Abdominal complications:**
  - Ileus:
    - Presents with abdominal distention, discomfort, and decreased flatulence.
    - Treatment:
      ○ Place patients NPO, administer intravenous fluids and bowel rest.
      ○ Liberal use of laxatives and slow diet advancement when symptoms resolve.
- Ureteral injury
    - Occurs during deep dissection adjacent to the disk space.
    - Prevent by identification in the surgical field and lateral retraction.
  - Hernia:
    - Caused by improper closure of fascial layers.
- **Subsidence/end plate fracture, graft dislodgement:**
  - Caused by improper cage placement and sizing.
  - Presents with retropulsed fragments, neuroforaminal impingement, and pseudoarthrosis.
  - Prevention:
    - Appropriate preoperative imaging to ensure proper surgical approach.
    - Maintenance of midline orientation via fluoroscopic imaging.
    - Appropriate testing of implant sizes intraoperatively.

■ Suggested Readings

1. Sasso RC, Kenneth Burkus J, LeHuec JC. Retrograde ejaculation after anterior lumbar interbody fusion: transperitoneal versus retroperitoneal exposure. Spine 2003;28(10):1023–1026, 2010, 35, E622

2. Than KD, Wang AC, Rahman SU, et al. Complication avoidance and management in anterior lumbar interbody fusion. Neurosurg Focus 2011;31(4):E6

3. Tiusanen H, Seitsalo S, Osterman K, Soini J. Retrograde ejaculation after anterior interbody lumbar fusion. Eur Spine J 1995;4(6):339–342